Pure Life

Pure Life

✦

The Pura Vida Journey

Dr. Suzanne Osborne

iUniverse, Inc.
New York Lincoln Shanghai

Pure Life
The Pura Vida Journey

Copyright © 2007, 2008 by Dr. Suzanne Osborne

iUniverse books may be ordered through booksellers or by contacting:

iUniverse
2021 Pine Lake Road, Suite 100
Lincoln, NE 68512
www.iuniverse.com
1-800-Authors (1-800-288-4677)

Because of the dynamic nature of the Internet, any Web addresses or links contained in this book may have changed since publication and may no longer be valid.

The information, ideas, and suggestions in this book are not intended as a substitute for professional medical advice. Before following any suggestions contained in this book, you should consult your personal physician. Neither the author nor the publisher shall be liable or responsible for any loss or damage allegedly arising as a consequence of your use or application of any information or suggestions in this book.

ISBN: 978-0-595-45484-6 (pbk)
ISBN: 978-0-595-69687-1 (cloth)
ISBN: 978-0-595-89796-4 (ebk)

Printed in the United States of America

Dedication: To Orianna

At a unique health food restaurant nestled deep in the lush jungle bordering Costa Rica's Monteverde Reserve, my husband Len and I met a special child who enriched our lives and helped us see the world through changed eyes. She was a radiant, thoughtful little girl, whose name, Orianna (which means Golden One) matched her lively personality.

As the daughter of a local Quaker guide and a nurturing, artistic mother, Orianna was raised in the unspoiled, protected wilderness at the edge of a misty cloudforest. Wise beyond her years, this angelic eight-year-old passionately related the plight of the rainforest as she led us through the dappled light of the jungle on muddy afternoon walks.

Through this poster child for healthy living, our awareness of certain aspects of nature—such as identifying the songs of brightly colored birds and locating endangered golden beetles and other crawly creatures—was greatly heightened. When I write about Pure Life and remembering what it was like to be a child, being active, and moving for the sake of movement, I often think of Orianna.

On one magical, moonlit evening at a musical gathering in the cloudforest restaurant, she expressed her zest for life in a way that only she could. After the native guitar and harmonica players shared their lively music with the crowd, some local musicians discovered a hauntingly soothing, hypnotic tempo on a variety of large percussion instruments, producing a deep, resonating sound reminiscent of an African tribal campfire.

While enjoying the primeval drumming, several of us moved to the wooden porch to stargaze and enjoy the crisp night air. From there we witnessed a touching sight in the yard below that I will never forget—Orianna, with her golden hair illuminated by the light of the full moon and a tiny campfire, dancing joyfully in synch with the ancient tempo, uniquely expressing her gift of freedom and life with pure joy and uninhibited laughter.

As it has since the dawn of humanity, the power of rhythm moved her, and in turn, each of us. It seemed that we were each acutely aware of the rhythm of the drums and for just a moment, I could vividly remember what it felt like to be a child growing up in the mountains of West Virginia, playing, laughing, and running so hard that I often had to stop to catch my breath.

Orianna dancing was truly a Pure Life moment, connecting and uniting people from all over the world who had just met. Her youthful, free-spirited exuberance energized and inspired us all and made each of us feel connected, both to each other and to the vibrant, youthful energy of the entire universe.

I often think of Orianna when I am simply cutting loose and doing something purely spontaneous—just for the fun of it. She reminded me that I do not always have to move in a structured world of rules and regulations, and that life is meant to be lived fully and in the moment.

Like children all over the world, Orianna was not afraid to seize the moment and totally immersed herself in the experience of living. We adults can all learn valuable, life changing lessons from these little people, if only we take time to listen to them and allow them to teach us.

I feel blessed to have spent time with this innocent and inspirational child who truly cared about the fragile ecosystems of the rainforest in a heart-felt, personal way that is difficult for most of us to imagine. In turn, the rainforest and its shy inhabitants revealed their ancient secrets to her. Thank you Orianna, wherever you are, for sharing your special world with us, and for inspiring me to share my words and experiences with others.

Contents

Preface ix

Introduction xiii

Pure Energy 1

The Power of Visualization 6

Remaining Calm In The Concrete Jungle 15

The Breath Of Life 22

Meditation 28

Positive Body Image 32

Strong, Confident, Healthy Posture 36

The Truth About Excess Bodyfat 40

Pure H$_2$O 45

Eating For Content 50

Why Diets Simply Do Not Work 53

Pure Fuel 56

Fiber And Whole Foods 61

Complex Carbohydrates: Pure Energy Fuel 66

Pure Protein 73

The Truth About Dietary Fats 76

Reflective Interlude 83

The Transition Stage 87

Dietary Fat Reduction Tips 92

Sodium Balance 101

Nutrition And Supplementation 104

Vitamins 111

Minerals From The Earth 115

Mother Nature's Secrets 120

Women And Excess Bodyfat 124

The Power Of Exercise 137

Feeling Stronger Every Day 145

Stretching For Health 151

Exercising Aerobically 156

Walking For Life 164

Muscle Anatomy 166

Strength Training With Weights 173

Weight Training Exercises That Work 181

Dangerous Exercises 194

On the Road 197

Practical Advice 200

Creating Health 211

Pura Vida! 216

The Pure Life Stepping Stones 219

Preface

The native Costa Ricans have a lovely saying that is truly symbolic of their unique way of living: *Pura Vida*, which literally means Pure Life. It is used as a warm, friendly greeting, and as an expression of the inner joy that they feel while living their simple, natural lives—one day at a time.

The natives, or *Ticos*, have an almost childlike zest for life and take time to fully appreciate and thoroughly enjoy life's simple pleasures. Their Pura Vida philosophy was the inspiration for this book.

Like millions of others, my husband Len and I have always been drawn to the primal energy and raw, quiet beauty of rainforests. Eventually, our journey through life led us to the Monteverde Biological Reserve in Costa Rica, one of the last remaining virgin cloudforests in the world. Here, for an entire month on two separate occasions in the early nineties, we were able to temporarily leave behind our busy, often hectic lives, and concentrate on taking time to collect our thoughts, while living completely and fully in the moment.

Together, we experienced the exhilarating feeling that comes from breathing fresh, unpolluted, oxygen-rich air as we hiked under the canopies of ancient strangler fig trees. In the jungle bordering the mountaintop village of Monteverde, we experienced the true meaning of the Pura Vida philosophy while galloping high-spirited horses along the ridges of lush, green volcanic mountain ranges.

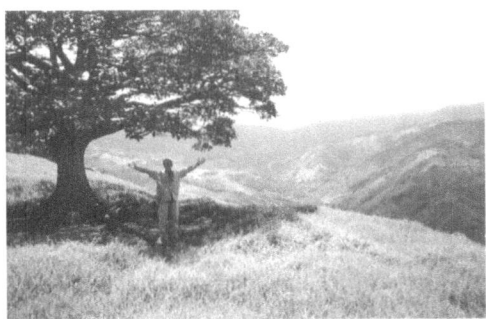

From its beginning, our journey seemed to be propelled and guided by a series of meaningful coincidences, with one helpful person leading to another, charting the course for an adventure that eventually took on a slow, sensual rhythm of its own.

As our Pura Vida adventure progressed, we began to feel as if we were slowly moving back in time toward a simpler, more balanced, and healthier way of life. Certain areas seemed to possess an almost magical power to transport us to another place and time.

Clearly etched in my memory is the moment that we spotted a pair of brilliant, rare quetzal birds nesting near a pristine waterfall in the cloudforest. It truly felt as though time were standing still as we watched these exotic, iridescent, blue-green and crimson creatures with tail feathers close to two feet long, fluttering gracefully in one of their last refuges on earth.

I will never forget the feeling of the powerful, primordial energy of ten-foot waves crashing over us while body-surfing along the rugged shores of Montezuma (a wild, frontier-like town on the Gulf of Nicoya).

I will always treasure my memories of the humble, gentle people that we met in Costa Rica who changed our lives for the better and reminded us just how closely interconnected and integrally related we all are to each other and to our environment.

Our adventures and experiences in Costa Rica also helped to reaffirm our belief in the interconnection between the spiritual mind and the physical body, and the power of one to affect the other. It was during this time in the jungle that I felt compelled to begin organizing and condensing the health related information and ideas that I have collected over the course of two decades.

The end result is the book that you are holding. I sincerely hope that you will gain some useful insight from reading it and referring back to it as your personal guidebook for healthier, stronger, and more energetic living.

One of my most firmly held personal beliefs is that our inner energy is our greatest resource and that when we are in touch with this energy, we have the power to change our lives for the better. I also believe that one's mind, body, and spirit must be in balanced harmony in order to realize a life filled with maximum, pure energy.

As a retired doctor of chiropractic and active holistic health and fitness educator who has treated thousands of patients since 1986, I have found that the more I study subjects such as neural anatomy, exercise physiology, and nutrition, the more respect I have for my own body, and, in turn, for its creator. I have been fascinated with the intricate workings of the human body since childhood, and never cease to be amazed by the power of the body to heal itself under the proper conditions.

In writing this book my intention is to share valuable, practical information and advice that will help you create a solid foundation on which to build your own uniquely healthy and energetic lifestyle, and also to discover the extraordinary potential that lies deep within you.

Knowledge truly is power, and learning is a never-ending process that is affected by our constantly evolving belief systems and life experiences. What is presently accepted as common knowledge or scientific fact will change drastically in a few years. What will not change, however, is the basic concept of treating your body with the respect it deserves, ultimately improving the quality of your life and your spiritual and emotional well-being.

Understandably, not everyone will agree with or relate to what I have to share in this book. What really matters is that you come away with some positive information and ideas that will improve or transform your present lifestyle, and enrich your everyday life experiences. My goal in writing this book is to provide you with a unique, fresh perspective on optimal health and motivate you to take the necessary steps to change your life for the better.

The Pure Life philosophy is not a rigid, perfectionist, or obsessive way of living, but rather a powerful feeling of being full of life and energy. The title of this book was inspired by a meaningful experience that we shared with our Costa Rican amigo, *Abuelo* (Spanish for grandfather) during one misty morning at our rainforest lodge.

As we watched Abuelo effortlessly cutting acres of green grass with a machete, Len and I asked him where he found the energy to basically mow the lawn with a machete, day after day.

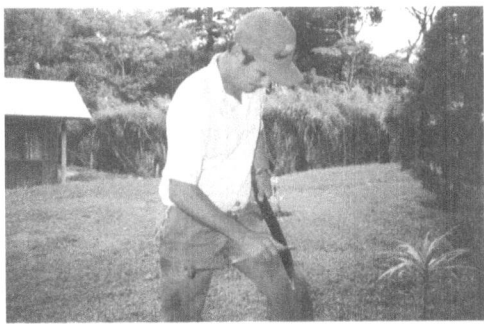

He simply smiled, took a deep breath of fresh air, and raised his outstretched arms toward the rising sun, joyfully answering "Pura Vida!" It was a simple, yet meaningful moment that touched us deeply.

Thank you for keeping an open mind and for choosing to be a part of the grassroots Pura Vida Movement by reading this book. As you travel along your unique path, remember to focus on the positive aspects of your life, be grateful for the little things, and take time to take care of yourself. Perhaps most importantly, make it a point to have fun and thoroughly enjoy the precious gift of life itself.

Buena suerte (good luck) on your own exhilarating Pure Life journey.
Dr. Suzy (Your Pura Vida Guide)

Introduction

The state of your health at this precise moment is a reflection of every choice you have ever made in your entire life. In other words, your health is a direct result of the decisions that you make on a daily basis.

Enjoying optimal health is an ongoing process, a way of life that gradually unfolds and evolves, not a quick six or twelve week program. True health is not an actual destination but rather an exciting journey of personal growth and discovery, encompassing the synchronous voyages of the body, mind, and soul.

I have found that navigating my own life course and deciding which path to take is much easier when I slow down and take time to listen to my own inner guidance, allowing my mind to function intuitively. This valuable lesson was reinforced many times during our life affirming adventures in Costa Rica.

At the beginning of our travels, still somewhat wired from our busy cyberworld, Len and I found that when we tried to strategically plan our days and demanded an exact time frame from the Ticos, they looked at us with a knowing smile and often repeated the word *tranquilo* (meaning tranquil or calm).

We soon learned that if we simply relaxed and went with the natural flow of events, something unexpected usually happened, which was much more interesting and exciting than whatever we were attempting to force to happen within our rigid time frame.

For example, applying the lesson of *Tranquilo* and following our instincts led us to a rustic sign for homemade oatmeal cookies at the end of an extremely long, dusty, and bumpy road in Monteverde. This sign, in turn, led us to our good friend Tony Nunnery, the most knowledgeable and intuitive guide in Costa Rica.

As a bilingual schoolteacher who had walked from Texas to Central America—leaving behind most of his possessions—Tony was a gold mine of information about Costa Rica and life in general.

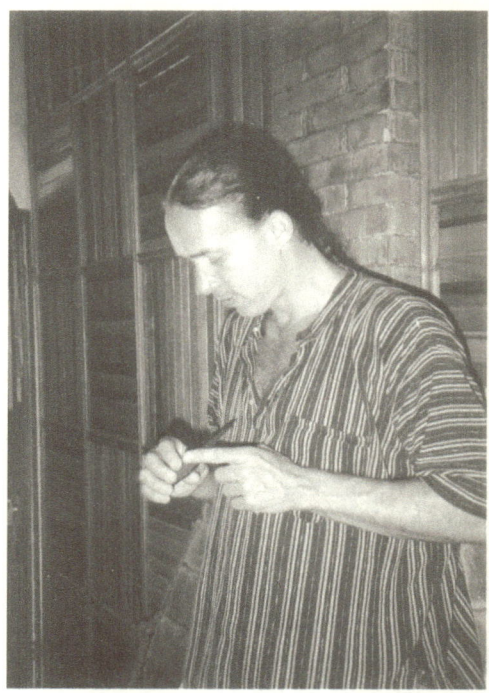

From his former National Geographic photographer's hideout deep in the jungle, he led us across the country to wild, magical places that we may never have discovered if we had not taken a chance and followed our intuition and the meaningful signs along the way.

During this time, we also found that an event that we would normally perceive as an inconvenience or delay often turned out to be a rerouting opportunity which led us to another truly meaningful experience or valuable life lesson.

As you have traveled on your own unique journey through life, you have also experienced surprising connections or meaningful coincidences that led you on to exciting new pathways. As your Pura Vida guide, I trust that after reading this book, you will discover some information or ideas that will help you chose the right turn at precisely the right time, and provide you with a clearer sense of direction and purpose in life.

When it comes to your own health, most of the time—deep down—you instinctively know what the right choice is. The challenge that we all face is having the willpower to make the right decision and ultimately follow the path that is best for us.

When you slow down and take time to ask yourself, "What are the health consequences of this choice that I am making?" it is much easier to hear what your inner voice is trying to tell you. It is important to remember that it is not what you do occasionally that makes you healthy, but rather, what you do consistently. Also, simply knowing that you *should* do something does not have the same power as knowing *why* you should do it.

Once an individual gains a clearer understanding of exactly *why* it is so important to take care of their body and nourish their soul, it is much easier for them to make necessary lifestyle changes. There is a certain level of calm, quiet strength that can be obtained as a result of positive change, which provides a healthy Pure Life Momentum and makes it easier for each of us to continue along the right path.

Pure Life is not another miracle diet book written by a famous celebrity or supermodel. Nor is it a trendy program created by experienced marketing specialists. This book was written by a real person with the help of her very supportive and patient husband. Although we have had some very unique experiences, Len and I live relatively normal lives, perhaps much like yours. Also, like you, we are constantly evolving and changing as we live each day, hopefully learning from our mistakes and experiences.

Living a consistently healthy lifestyle has always been a high priority in both of our lives; however, our personal voyage of optimal health and wellness has not always been one of perfectly smooth sailing. There have been numerous obstacles, sudden storms, and unexpected detours along the way, each offering its own unique combination of learning opportunities.

One thing that I personally have found particularly challenging through the years is deciding exactly who and what to believe, especially when advising patients. As you have undoubtedly found, it is often difficult to extract the truth hidden in the labyrinth of conflicting information available today.

Unlike many experts of every sort, celebrities, and gurus who churn out best sellers about health under pressing deadlines, I have taken my own sweet, *tranquilo* time to write this book, fully living, working, and practicing what I have written during the entire process.

My personal journey has included over twenty years of research, not only through schools of higher education, books, periodicals, and seminars, but perhaps more importantly, through practical research and application, often learning the hard way, through trial and error and life experience.

Rather than simply adding to the confusion and controversy surrounding many health related subjects, I have focused on providing you with the simple basics; practical information that will aid you in making daily decisions about your health and help you form your own unique personal health belief system.

One of my primary reasons for writing this book was to answer some of the hundreds of sincere questions that I have been asked by my patients, consulting clients, online and magazine readers, friends, and family over the years.

In fact, some of the text in this book was written as early as 1986 in response to specific questions that some of my inquisitive patients asked. At that time, I could never have dreamed that someday in the future, I would access unlimited volumes of information and research from the internet in a matter of seconds.

Neither could I have imagined that we would create an information based website (www.pure-life.com) that would be visited by millions of people from every corner of the world and make it possible for me to achieve my goal of sharing what I have learned with others on a global scale.

When we first launched the website in 1995, the internet was still a somewhat mysterious concept to most Americans and many thought that it wouldn't last. I can remember people looking at my like I was from another planet when I first mentioned the word blog.

Pure-life.com started as a simple, question and answer reference library of information that was disseminated gradually over the years. It first gained popularity with online visitors interested in Costa Rica, and quickly evolved into a widely recognized source for holistic and alternative health information and advice.

Around 2004, the site grew to include an internet based retail store, offering a wide variety of products that we have found to be safe and effective. During those years, I learned a great deal about natural health care products and received invaluable information and unbiased testimonials related to pain relief, stress reduction, and wellness products.

I continue to share honest feedback about helpful products both on the site and also throughout this book. In Chapter 36 of this book, I highlight a few of my all time favorite wellness products and share practical advice that can make a dramatic difference in the quality of your daily life.

In recent years, pure-life.com has returned to its more simple roots and currently focuses primarily on education. The site contains various health related articles that I have written for national magazines and information that serves as an adjunct to this book, such as a downloadable version of the stretching method that I developed and now teach to others.

The content of pure-life.com is constantly evolving and changing in an effort to be current and relative to what is going on in the world at that particular time.

The basic mission of the site and the book remains the same, however: to help individuals create healthier, stronger and more energetically balanced lifestyles, one step at a time.

In collecting information for this book, I have often been motivated by patients from my chiropractic practice who were on their own truth-seeking journey. A large percentage of the content you'll read was inspired by their unique questions, heartfelt stories, and practical life experiences.

After providing health care to thousands of patients and advising them individually for more than ten years, I decided to share what I have learned from my experiences with as many people as possible through this book and related projects.

Considering how integrally related every subject concerning health truly is, I sometimes found it difficult to simply answer specific questions without trying to help the truth seeker see what I call the entire Pura Vida picture.

In writing this book, I soon realized that it is impossible to thoroughly cover every single subject of popular interest. So, instead, I decided to focus on what I truly believe in and what really works for me. What I have to share with you is what I have found to be true after weeding through everything I could get my hands on concerning holistic health, nutrition, and fitness, and consistently applying it in my daily life.

Instead of reading this book in the traditional way, I invite you to read slowly, taking your own *Tranquilo* time to apply what you are learning on a daily basis. Give the material plenty of time to soak into the fabric of your daily lifestyle. You will find plenty of statistics, facts and numbers laced throughout this book, but if you are anything like me, memorizing them doesn't always come easy. Fortunately, memorization of all the various facts and statistics isn't absolutely necessary and is a feat that I still haven't mastered after all of these years.

As with most things in life, the answers to the questions you may be seeking are usually not black and white. For this reason, I encourage you to do further research on your own on a continual basis, and gradually integrate the new information and concepts into your daily lifestyle. You will find that it can be extremely rewarding to research a particular subject and slowly discover your own truth.

I have always believed that true health consists of a healthy balance of the body, mind, and soul—what I like to call the Pure Life Triune. Since the soul is an integral component of this triune, I find it impossible to write about optimal health without first recognizing the vital importance of certain spiritual aspects, such as religious belief, faith, and love.

Clinical experience has led me to believe that a person's spiritual beliefs—regardless of whether they believe in Jesus, Buddha, a universal spirit, a higher power, etc.—have a direct impact on the state of their health and well being.

My husband and I have been extremely blessed, not only with a loving, healthy relationship, but also with a circle of close family and friends who are a vital, intrinsic part of our Pura Vida lifestyle.

As you have found on your own personal journey, every person's life touches that of others, interconnecting and affecting us all. The people that we meet and the valuable lessons that we have all learned along the way help form our spiritual beliefs and affect the way that we view the world and our place in it.

As you embark on your own Pura Vida adventure, I encourage you to not only feed your mind with powerful knowledge and move your body with strengthening exercise and physical activity, but also to nourish your soul, connecting with and awakening the pure life spirit within you.

As your Pura Vida guide, I will be there along the path to help clear the way, point out areas of danger and interest, and lend a helping hand if needed. Only you, however, have the power to make your journey a life altering voyage of personal discovery and pure energy.

Only you have the ability to create a permanently healthy, happy lifestyle. It is your life. Live it with intention and as if this moment is all there is!

Pure Energy

There is an awesome energy flowing deep inside of every one of us. It is the powerful, mysterious life force that coordinates and controls every function of our bodies, from the intricate process that naturally heals damaged tissues, to the automatic, rhythmic beating of our hearts approximately one hundred thousand times a day.

The ancient Greeks, and even one of my own personal heroes, Albert Einstein, were intrigued by this flow of energy or life force, just as we are today. The fascinating science of quantum physics has proven that bundles of this vibrating energy are constantly swirling at lightning speed through the vast empty space of the atoms that make up our physical bodies.

This inner energy goes by several names in many different languages. The yogis of ancient India called this vital life force *prana* and considered breathing to be the vehicle of *prana*. Throughout the centuries, Indian yogis have taught that controlling the breath controls the universal energy within, which directly affects one's physical health and state of mind.

Thousands of years ago, the Taoist sages of ancient China named this inner energy *qi*. Those who study Eastern philosophies believe that *qi*, (also known as *ki* and more commonly as *chi*) flows through several distinct pathways in the body, linking tissues, organs, and brain function into a unified whole.

They also believe that *qi* connects each person to the environment and, ultimately, to the entire universe. In essence, they feel that the primary energy of life found in the wind rustling through the leaves of the trees and in each fresh blade of grass growing on the earth, is the same universal energy that flows throughout our own bodies.

One of the basic tenets of Eastern philosophy involves the ancient law of interrelatedness, which basically states that nothing can exist in and of itself—that everything in the universe exists in relation to everything else.

Followers of ancient Eastern philosophy also believe that true health requires a delicate balance of two interdependent forces: *yin* and *yang*, which continually work to control, harmonize, and balance each other. In perfect alignment with the law of interrelatedness, these two forces are flowing and interdependent, not conflicting and opposed, as is commonly believed.

The *yin* phase of energy is associated with receptive, contractive characteristics and is present in such qualities as rest and passivity. The expansive, outgoing aspect of *yang* is present in such qualities as activity and stimulation. You do not have to look far to find examples of this concept in your everyday life; the contraction and relaxing of your muscles as you move, or a sudden burst of emotion followed by a sense of calm.

According to ancient Chinese tradition, the continual flow of *qi* through the dynamic forces of *yin* and *yang* is necessary to sustain life. It is also believed that a disharmony or lack of balance between these two aspects results in disease, or what is sometimes known in alternative healing as *dis-ease*, because the body is in a state which is the polar opposite of ease.

Most Eastern health care practitioners believe that there is a highly organized energy system in the body, completely separate and distinct from the nervous system, but running along similar pathways.

After scientifically observing living human beings throughout the centuries, Eastern medicine has established precise and orderly patterns, called meridians, through which practitioners believe this energy, or life force, flows.

Conventional Western medicine, on the other hand, has resisted accepting the existence of such a system, and, until recently, has viewed the body as basically a machine that is kept running by some mysterious, unknowable force, that can be neither measured nor seen.

The old Western medical paradigm was based largely on the study of lifeless human bodies and had a tendency to view the human body as a chemical machine composed of highly specialized parts. Fortunately, this view is gradually being replaced with a new model, which focuses on the interconnectedness of the human body, mind, and spirit—the Pure Life Triune.

This new alternative approach to health care is actually ancient in that it draws from the healing wisdom of a variety of cultures—some over ten thousand years old—and also from alternative holistic health care systems, such as Ayurvedic and Chinese medicine, Homeopathy, Chiropractic, and Naturopathy.

The philosophies which comprise the foundation of these alternative health care systems are similar in that they tend to view each part of the body not only in terms of how that particular organ or part functions on its own, but rather in terms of its role in relation to the entire system or the whole person—hence the term Holistic.

Throughout history, holistic health care practitioners have been trained to view the patient as a whole, complete physical, mental, and spiritual being, rather than simply the gallbladder patient in room 404.

Although the term alternative medicine has gradually seeped into our society's current vocabulary, I prefer to use terms such as alternative to medicine and alternative or holistic health care systems.

I also find it very interesting that after many years of criticizing and ridiculing alternative health care providers, the medical profession has recently begun absorbing various aspects of these now popular alternative methods and techniques into their own traditional medical practices.

In the interest of fairness, conventional Western medicine has an important place in the broad spectrum of health care systems and many of us would not be alive today without drugs or surgery. Some of the recent technological advances made in modern medicine are truly remarkable.

In fact, much of the scientific information that I am sharing with you in this book is the result of dedicated professionals working diligently in this area. Some of my most open-minded patients have been hard working medical doctors, nurses, and others involved in traditional medical professions.

I do believe that traditional Western medicine as a whole, however, could benefit tremendously by spending more time looking at the other half of the health care picture. True health care includes recognizing the vital importance of maintaining a harmonious, healthy balance between the body, mind, and soul, and acknowledging the existence of an inner energy that does more than simply keep the physical body running.

As Thomas Edison once said, "The doctor of the future will give no medicine, but will interest his patients in the care of the human frame, in diet, and in the cause and prevention of disease." To me, this is an extremely powerful statement, especially considering that the word doctor originally comes from a Latin word meaning teacher. As I experienced firsthand in my own clinical practice, there is little time for patient education and training in today's managed health care system.

Fortunately, in the past decade or so, there has been a dramatic shift toward holistic health care systems that offer a more integrated approach, treating the whole person rather than focusing solely on isolated symptoms or specific body parts.

This positive change is due largely to the increased awareness of individuals who are beginning to take a more active role in their own health care, and seeking ways other than drugs and surgery to maintain health and prevent disease. People are finally taking more responsibility for their own health and well-being and are no longer voiceless, passive participants in determining the future direction of their own health care.

Like many people throughout the world, I firmly believe that energy is the basis of all life and that the free flow of this energy is directly related to the state of one's health. I also believe that there is an inborn or innate intelligence in the human body that is responsible for organizing and directing the flow of this energy throughout all of its systems.

Like a starfish that possesses the innate ability to regrow a lost limb, your body is truly amazing in that it has the ability to heal itself. You need only to witness the miraculous transformation of a superficial cut on the skin into healthy new living tissue to demonstrate this fact.

The human body is dynamic and is continuously changing. Your body is constantly rebuilding and renewing itself—a truly miraculous work of art in progress. You shed millions of skin cells a day, your liver replaces itself every six weeks, and you obtain a new stomach lining every five days.

The living tissue of your bones is constantly being broken down and rebuilt. In a young person, old bone is replaced by new bone every ninety days. In essence, you are actually a different person today than you were yesterday.

It is the natural condition of the human body to be healthy, just as it is natural for a bird to fly or a tree to grow. Like any other living organism, however, your body can only be healthy under the right conditions. Your body has specific needs, such as fresh air, pure water, nutritious food, and physical activity, which must be met in order for it to remain healthy and to thrive.

Lately, we frequently hear the word health in conversation and in the media: i.e. health and fitness, health care, healthy products, etc. Few of us have ever stopped and considered the true meaning of the word, however.

True health is not about simply looking healthy and attractive on the outside or having a perfect, rock hard body. Health does not come in a bottle. Optimal health comes from the inside, and is not merely the absence of disease or symptoms, just as light is not simply the absence of darkness.

Pure health is something in and of itself—an optimum state of physical, mental, spiritual, and even social well-being. It is a union of many different parts that are all necessary to make up the balanced whole. For this reason, you cannot simply change one aspect of your lifestyle in order to achieve optimal health, if other areas of your life are not properly balanced.

In the words of Hippocrates "A wise man ought to realize that health is his most valuable possession." Accumulating a vast amount of money, status, or expensive objects means nothing, if it is gained at the expense of your physical health or emotional well-being. We all have the potential to be healthier. It is simply a matter of making our health a very high priority in our lives. With this in mind, this book was written as a practical guidebook for people who want to take an active role in establishing the healthy lifestyle of which they have always dreamed.

We all pass through different stages in our own personal journeys of optimal health. You will notice that a great deal of the information and suggestions that I am sharing with you is directed toward individuals who are just beginning to make healthy lifestyle changes.

Regardless of the level of health that you have already achieved in your daily lifestyle, however, I trust that you will find some valuable information that will help you improve the quality of your life and increase your pure energy level.

The most common question that people have asked me over the years is basically this: "How long will it take?" The answer is usually simple: "The rest of your life." You are going to live in the same body that you inhabit now for all of your remaining days on this earth.

You cannot buy a brand new body when this one wears out. You cannot trade it in on a newer, shinier model, or order all new replacement parts. That is exactly why it is so important to start treating your body with the respect it deserves right now—not some magical, perfect day in the future that, inevitably, never comes.

Regardless of your past history, you can begin your personal Pura Vida journey of permanent optimal health at this very moment simply by making the decision to create a higher state of health and a more joyful, balanced life. It is never too late to start feeling stronger and more confident. It is never too late to start becoming the truly healthy person that you have always dreamed of being. The choice is yours to make.

As you continue reading this book and traveling on your unique path, please keep the following word in mind: *awareness*. Whether we are discussing deep breathing, nutrition, posture, stretching, or any other health related topic, becoming more aware will make you feel more alive in the present moment and improve your odds of successfully achieving the lifestyle you deserve.

The Power of Visualization

o o o o o o o o o o o o o o o o o o o o o o o o o o o o o o o o o o o o o
Those who contemplate the beauty of the earth find reserves of strength that will endure as long as life lasts.

—*Rachel Carson*

As you embark on your own unique Pura Vida journey, I encourage you to take time to practice using the awesome power of creative visualization on a regular basis. By tapping into the endless resources of your imagination, visualization can help you to reduce your stress level, induce a state of deep relaxation, and achieve goals that you may have never dreamed were possible.

By combining visualization with meditation techniques, you can effectively use the creative power of your mind to actually see the direction in which you want your personal journey through life to proceed, from this moment on.

According to many highly respected research scientists, doctors, and quantum physicists, changing the way that we think creates a quantum field of possibilities that can positively affect the outcome of our day, and eventually change the course of our lives. Put quite simply, we basically become what we think about all day.

Research shows that over time, thinking the same thought repeatedly creates a solid neural pathway that becomes part of the operational software of our brain. For example, if we repeatedly think that we are fat or unhealthy, then eventually we come to believe that as our current reality and each time we hear that old negative script in our head, we are reinforcing and strengthening our brain's own unique circuitry.

Over time, our brain creates something called a neuro-net, which is basically an immensely complicated network within our brains that interconnects the nerve cells at junctions called synapses. Unfortunately, it seems that most of us are running on old, outdated operational software for our brains and don't utilize a very large percentage of what brainpower we have.

Scientists know about this phenomenon because even though they cannot see the actual junction where the neural impulses connect, they can measure the electrical activity in the brain. Using technologically advanced tools such as PET scanning imagery, scientists can see the little lightning storms that go off in different parts of our brain depending and what we are seeing, experiencing, and thinking.

Our amazing body also produces chemicals as a result of thoughts. If you think about something that makes you extremely stressed, for example, your body releases the hormone cortisol. Thinking the same stressful thought over and over reinforces the neural pathways of your brain and becomes an integral part of the operational software of your brain, as well.

Fortunately, thinking fresh, new thoughts about abstract future possibilities actually stimulates new growth in your neural pathway structure and stimulates different, newer parts of the brain. Feel-good chemicals are also released when we repeatedly think about positive emotions such as love, establishing new pathways and networks.

Fortunately, we can actually upgrade our brain's operational software by thinking positive thoughts, such as those related to health, happiness, and success, establishing new pathways that create new realities and possibilities for us in the future.

I have experienced this phenomenon personally on many different occasions since beginning my first Chiropractic practice. I particularly enjoy observing how positive thinking and visualization make such a dramatic difference in the healing potential of various individuals. Those who believe that they will get well, often do. Those who believe that they have no part in the outcome have lower recovery rates as well.

It's all very deep and fascinating stuff. To me, the most amazing, yet mysterious part of all is that our bodies are actually composed of mostly empty matter swirling in space. The fact that the chair that you are sitting in isn't really, truly solid is a hard concept to swallow, I know. But when you look at everything on a subatomic or quantum level, the particles inside the atom only occupy a minute percentage of the overall space inside the atom. The rest of the vast inner space of the atom is largely occupied by bundles of vibrating matter or basically energy.

Yes, we are our bodies, but we are also the cumulative result of our cells on a molecular level. To put it simply, healthy cells mean a healthier body. That's why factors such as taking antioxidants and drinking water affect our health. They positively affect our cells, which improves our overall health and well being. It's also interesting to think about what happens when our cells divide and how they will carry the effects of our old way of thinking with them when they form the new structures of our bodies.

Thinking negative thoughts not only reinforces the old pathways but also affects us on a cellular level. If we truly believe that we can get a better job, get strong and healthy, or become financially successful, then we are creating new circuitry for our brains to run on. The really interesting part is that this new circuitry can create new possibilities and potential in our daily lives and increase the odds of achieving the goals we desire.

For many people, the most effective way to establish this new neural circuitry is through the regular practice of meditation. Like everything else that is worth doing in life, meditation takes time and practice. Once you begin fully integrating meditation into your daily lifestyle, however, you will not only achieve a heightened state of awareness and increased energy, but you will also benefit even more from the productive practice of creative visualization.

When you have the time and opportunity, you can begin the creative visualization process by simply imagining yourself in an environment that you associate with relaxing—one in which you feel at peace, yet fully alive. Close your eyes and visualize yourself relaxing at your favorite beach, on top of a familiar mountain, beside a gentle, soothing stream or a magnificent waterfall—any special spot, real or imaginary, where you feel safe, relaxed, and full of positive energy.

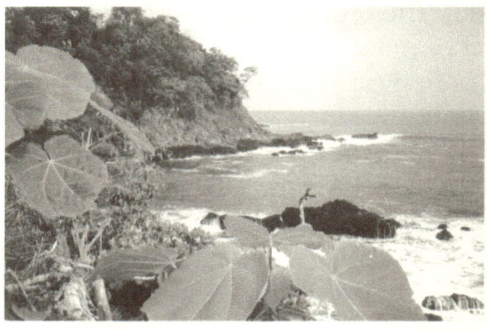

Then, take long, slow, deep breaths—vividly imagining the sights, sounds, and smells—as you focus on creating a fertile oasis of *tranquilo* that you can return to again and again, regardless of the everyday distractions surrounding you. As you concentrate on your breathing, take some time to evaluate your overall lifestyle exactly as it is at this moment. Take a good, long look inward and be totally honest with yourself.

Then, visualize what you want to accomplish, and how you would like to look and feel in the near future. If you have a specific goal such as running a marathon, or living to see your grandchildren have children, focus on the positive details of that goal. See yourself living a balanced life, filled with maximum energy and nurturing relationships. Picture yourself with crystal clear eyes, a healthy physique, and a radiant smile. Imagine yourself vibrant in your later years, pain and disease-free, enjoying your favorite activities and sharing your wisdom and experience with others.

Visualize yourself repeatedly making the right decisions along the path of optimal health. Spend a considerable amount of time visualizing the positive rewards—both physical and emotional—of making those decisions. Hold this image firm in your mind's eye. Repeat this practice as often as possible, preferably on a daily basis. It only takes a few minutes and is an excellent aid in reducing stress throughout your day.

Several images that I personally associate with my own visualizations and meditation are forever ingrained in my consciousness as part of our Costa Rican adventures. I invite you to take a few minutes to set aside your worries and forget about the practical concerns of the real world, as we travel together on an allegorical hike through your own Pura Vida rainforest.

Picture yourself walking along a lush, imaginary trail hidden deep in the cloudforest, dripping with luminous green vines, giant ferns, and fragile air plants. Visualize the dappled, golden light of the sun sparkling on the wings of brilliant, giant blue morpho butterflies and iridescent flowers.

As you picture yourself walking through the fresh, fragrant air, imagine a sapphire hummingbird hanging magically suspended in the air in front of you for several heart-stopping moments before buzzing on. See yourself hiking under the protective canopies of trees over a hundred feet tall, while families of lively howler monkeys playfully crash through the branches overhead. Hear the noisy squawking of green parrots and the joyful music of a variety of exotic birds and insects filling the air.

As you continue along your path, breathing in the rich, fresh, oxygen saturated air, you soon find that the trail—much like your journey of optimal health—has become a little more challenging and difficult when you least expected it.

As you continue upward on the increasingly steep, slippery trail, grabbing vines for support, you consider turning back, but then you discover something that encourages you to keep moving forward. Partially covered by the roots of the strangler fig trees growing like melted candle wax along the path, you find that someone has painstakingly placed large, sturdy stepping stones from an ancient river bed along the trail in front of you.

By utilizing these stepping stones, you are able to travel faster, farther, and higher than you originally thought possible. As you focus your energy on the challenging trail ahead of you, you realize that with the use of each stepping stone comes a greater sense of accomplishment and increased self-confidence.

As your heart pumps faster, circulating more oxygenated blood throughout your body, you feel ecstatically alive, much more so than you would on a well traveled, meandering trail. You gratefully acknowledge the soreness in your legs as a sign that your muscles are becoming stronger. With increased physical exertion comes increased strength and flexibility.

The path is becoming more challenging with every step, yet once you have experienced the satisfaction that results from reaching a higher level, it actually becomes easier for you to progress farther in the right direction. You are going with the natural flow of your body. The momentum of your pure energy carries you on to the next level.

Instead of rushing along the path, you decide to savor every moment, rewarding yourself by taking time to playfully swing from the vines along the less challenging areas and sit quietly on a moss-covered rock. Fully immersed in the feeling of *tranquilo*, you take time to soak your feet in the pools of a secret, multi-tiered waterfall plunging through the mystical cloudforest.

Relaxing and recharging in the sun, your mind wanders and you think about how many times in your life you have hurriedly pushed yourself along from one experience to another without stopping to enjoy your accomplishments along the way. You realize that the only person you have been racing with all this time is yourself. Vowing to learn from your experiences and also to give yourself credit when it is due, you continue along the steep path.

Refreshed and renewed, you tackle each difficult spot along the trail with the help of the ancient stepping stones, benefiting from the cumulative skill and knowledge gained as a result of your previous accomplishments.

As you confidently approach your intended destination (a sunlit peak with breathtaking panoramic views of other mountain ranges) you gain a fresh, new perspective and realize that this magnificent peak is but one of many. You now know that your journey has not ended, but is actually just beginning, continually unfolding and progressing to even higher, more awe inspiring levels.

With the help of the stepping stones, you were able to overcome seemingly insurmountable obstacles, learning and growing from each experience. Standing on top of the world with the energizing rays of the sun warming your shoulders, you enjoy a heightened sense of well being and clarity, and can actually feel the incredible magnetic pull of nature and sense the pulsing energy of the entire universe.

You allow yourself to fully enjoy this moment and, in doing so, you connect with the universal ebb and flow of life itself. Like our friend Abuelo, you raise your arms to the sky and shout "Pura Vida!" fully understanding the pure energy and zest for life behind his boyish enthusiasm.

As you travel farther on your Real Life Pura Vida journey, and continue reading this book, you will gradually discover sixteen ancient stepping stones at crucial points along your Pure Life path. These allegorical stepping stones have been strategically placed by other wise and helpful travelers over the course of thousands of years.

In many cases, their children have accompanied these travelers on their journey, and these sons and daughters have passed down the secret location of the stepping stones through successive generations, who have cleared away the inevitable, encroaching vines and debris so that you too, can benefit from taking these crucial steps toward a healthier, more energetic lifestyle.

There are countless branches and side trails off of the Pura Vida path, and each of us takes an entirely unique route. Eventually, however, we will all encounter areas where it is necessary to use the stepping stones to progress further.

Since positive change in any aspect of your life affects all other areas, you may adopt these stepping stones at any time you wish, and in any order you like. No one is more important than the others. Although adopting just one stepping stone will lead to improved health and increased energy, adopting all sixteen will lead to an expansion of pure energy and vitality that can radically improve your life.

A journey of a thousand miles starts with a single step, and you have already started the momentum rolling in the right direction. The simple fact that you chose to read this book shows that you have the desire to improve the quality of your health, and ultimately, your entire life. Fortunately, none of us has to be stuck in a comfortable rut unless we choose that path. We can each pull ourselves up by our own bootstraps, take charge of our destiny, and become our own mover and shaker.

Although other people can help motivate and inspire you, no one else can change your life for you. Here lies the simple secret: ultimately, you must do it for yourself, because you truly desire to permanently change your lifestyle for the better.

It is important to remember that positive changes do not usually take place overnight. Making noticeable changes in your way of living may seem challenging at first because your body may have become a little too comfortable and passive in its daily routine and it may initially resist active change.

In the beginning, your mind and soul may choose to take the higher path, yet your body may prefer to stay at home and camp out on the couch with a jumbo bag of potato chips and get lost in some mindless television program.

Creating a healthier, more energetic lifestyle sometimes requires a complete transformation in attitude in order to break the momentum of past habits. There are probably certain things you have always known that you should not do, but it is possible that you simply have not had the necessary, strong, disciplined mindset to change the unhealthy habits.

Positive change often involves the severing of intense emotional bonds to something that is holding you back. As you grow in awareness, you may find that certain aspects of your old conditioning must change. Sometimes, the path of right action and self-change involves a radical departure from old ways.

With the shedding of old habits, however, come powerful forces of change, liberating new energies that support a new way of being—a new way of living. Instead of searching for instant gratification, you will learn to concentrate on cultivating habits that leave you with a long-term sense of well-being and calm strength.

Never underestimate the power of your mind and will. Your good intentions and desires are actual positive forces that contain the unlimited potential power to transform your lifestyle. As your way of life is shifting and reforming, keep in mind that the new life is always greater than the old, and that new beginnings lead to renewed growth, new strength, and increased energy.

As you continue to evolve and your new life slowly unfolds, pay special attention to the intuitive side of your nature, and trust in the wisdom of instinct. Joyfully embrace positive change, remain receptive to new ideas and experiences, and do not be afraid to take chances every now and then.

The practice of letting the intuitive wisdom of your soul guide you, while simultaneously paying attention to what your body has to tell you, is so fundamental that the original seekers of truth along the Pure Life Journey made this principle the foundation for placing the first crucial stepping stone amidst the twisted vines of the Pura Vida path.

Since we are all not only biochemically, but spiritually and physiologically unique individuals, what is right for one of us is not necessarily right for all of us.

Consequently, the first crucial stepping stone on your Pure Life path is based on the wisdom of an ancient principle and is actually quite simple.

Stepping Stone # 1: *Listen closely to the innate intelligence of your body and let your intuitive nature guide you.*

For this powerful stepping stone, which also serves as a crucial touchstone, the Pura Vida path builders chose a massive, oval stone from an ancient riverbed. The surface of this giant stone has been worn smooth by centuries of nature's phenomenal forces flowing over it, gradually molding its unique shape and design. If you should find yourself veering too far off of the Pura Vida path and becoming frustrated or disoriented, you can always come back to this powerful touchstone to regain your focus and direction.

As members of our modern society, caught up in the sometimes frenetic swirl of everyday life, we are often too busy to recognize or actually choose to ignore the many warning signs and feedback that our bodies are constantly giving us.

When you eat a certain type of food and it causes indigestion or you experience pain in your back while lifting something that is too heavy, your body is desperately trying to tell you something. If you smelled smoke and heard your smoke detector, would you simply turn off the alarm and try to go back to sleep? Probably not. Yet, many of us choose to ignore obvious warning signs and symptoms relayed to us by the innate intelligence of our own bodies on a daily basis.

As I have personally witnessed numerous times during my years in practice, too often, it takes a serious or life threatening disease to make us stop and reevaluate our priorities or significantly change our lifestyles. The simple truth is that it takes effort and discipline to make major lifestyle changes, and moving steadily forward can sometimes be very challenging.

Of course, we all backslide at times, veering too far off onto the wrong trail, and eventually, we end up backtracking, losing valuable time and energy. These detours are a natural, integral part of the Pura Vida journey, however, and can serve as valuable learning experiences.

It is important to allow yourself room to make mistakes in your everyday life without feeling burdened by guilt. Do not be overly hard on yourself if you have temporarily fallen short of your goals or do not accomplish everything that you set out to do. Tomorrow is a new day, a fresh start, a clean slate.

In time, you can create and maintain the healthy balance that your body naturally desires by listening to your body's innate wisdom, which instinctively knows what is right for you. As you evolve and learn from your experiences, you will naturally make the choice that is ideal for you and become more determined not to slip backward or lose ground. The thought of eating one of your old unhealthy favorites, or lying around on the couch on a beautiful day, simply will not have the same appeal as it may have once had.

One of the truly beautiful benefits of adopting the Pura Vida philosophy is the positive effect it has on all other aspects of your life. Your relationships with family and friends automatically improve when you feel good about yourself and have achieved a more consistent, healthy level of energy. You may even serve as a source of inspiration to others without being aware of it.

In addition, your level of creativity and productivity naturally increases. Your career goals and purpose in life become clearer and more easily obtained as your health improves. You will find that it is much easier to flow with the natural course of life's peaks and valleys when your mind, body, and soul are in a harmonious balance.

Finally, you will experience the elusive feeling that many people seem to be searching for in all the wrong places. You will discover the inner joy and peace that comes from free, pure Pura Vida energy, direct from its natural source.

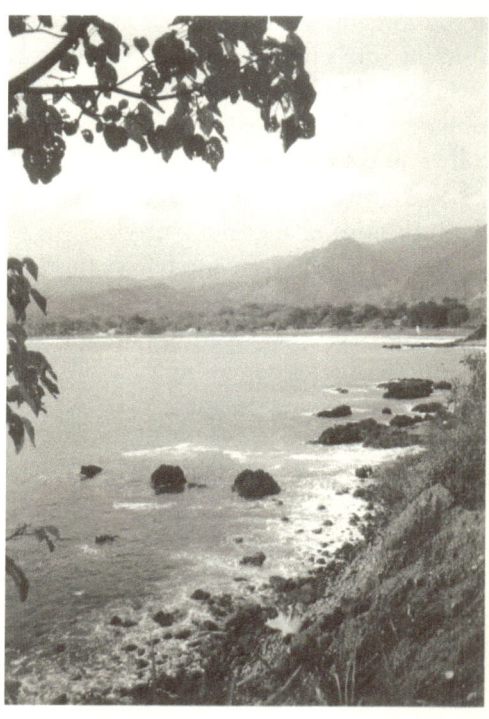

Remaining Calm In The Concrete Jungle

Len and I are firm believers in the power of positive thinking, and have seen the awesome effects of this philosophy demonstrated repeatedly in our own lives. It is our belief that the more energy you give something by thinking about it—regardless of whether the subject is positive or negative—the more you increase the odds of that particular event happening. Over time, whatever you focus your energy on will blossom, so be selective about what thoughts you allow into your mind.

Do not allow habitual, negative thoughts or old mental scripts to control your mind and determine your direction in life. Instead, write your own new Pure Life script, focus on the positive aspects of your life, and let your powerful mind guide your thoughts in a higher direction.

Perhaps Gandhi said it best: "*There is nothing more potent than thought. Deed follows word and word follows thought. The word is the result of a mighty thought, and where the thought is mighty and pure the result is always mighty and pure.*"

As a retired holistic health care practitioner and ongoing researcher of the truth as it relates to optimal health, I personally have come to believe that nothing has more power over your body than your mind. Consistent positive thinking can strengthen your immune system, reduce the negative effects of stress on your body, and considerably increase your pure energy level.

I have always found it amazing that until as recently as the sixties, many in the scientific community believed that our thoughts had no real, physical effect on our health; in essence, that the mind and body were separate entities.

Fortunately, what most of us have believed all along—that the mind, body, and soul are deeply interconnected—has now been scientifically proven and is widely accepted. Today, modern science has even coined a term (psychosomatic illness) for stress related conditions and diseases.

Continuous, overwhelming stress can be an insidious, silent killer. Stress is a leading contributor to coronary heart disease, which is the number one cause of death in America at this time, causing nearly half of all deaths in the United

States. Though cardiovascular disease has traditionally affected more males than females, it is now the number one killer of females in the U.S. as well.

According to Dr. Herbert Benson, a Harvard Medical School professor and founder of the Mind/Body Medical Institute, "70–90% of visits to the doctor are in the mind/body realm and are poorly served by drugs or surgery." Nevertheless, our society's dependence on over-the-counter and prescription drugs for psycho-somatic conditions is accelerating rapidly.

Like many others with alternative health care backgrounds, I am very alarmed by the sheer volume and presence of recent television, newspaper, and magazine advertisements seductively singing the praises of prescription drugs and recom-mending that you "Ask your doctor if a certain drug is right for you." It appears to me that as soon as a law was passed allowing the pharmaceutical industry to advertise on television, the advertising floodgates opened and the world has never been the same. We now know the names of prescription drugs that were previ-ously unheard of.

Through bombarding our collective subconscious with high budget, attrac-tive, psychologically manipulative ads, pharmaceutical companies are becoming increasingly richer and frighteningly powerful. In some cases, our society's stressed adults and impressionable children are being subliminally manipulated by faceless, politically powerful, billion dollar drug companies through ads such as these.

The long list of side effects, usually read in lengthy, yet reassuring, voiceovers (and sometimes taking up three-quarters of a page in printed ads) often include phrases such as: difficulty breathing and swallowing, heart attack, high blood pressure, intestinal bleeding, vomiting, kidney and liver damage, infection, pain, thoughts of suicide, and on and on. Pharmaceutical companies rely on funny and cute cartoon characters, beautiful scenery and computer generated imagery to sell their products. We have become so accustomed to hearing the lists of side effects that we subconsciously tune the majority of these disclaimers out without even realizing it.

Many people chose to believe that if a drug is approved by the F.D.A., then it must be safe. What most of us do not realize, however, is that certain dangerous side effects, sometimes including death, are not always evident in an approved drug until it has been taken by a large number of individuals in the general popu-lation over a lengthy period of time.

Throughout history, drugs that were touted upon their release as modern day miracles by the marketing experts of pharmaceutical companies have resulted in seriously harming trusting individuals who never questioned the possibility of negative side effects.

In today's rapidly paced world, some people simply find it easier to gamble on long term, detrimental side effects from taking prescription and over the counter drugs, rather than taking time to research or ask their doctor uncomfortable questions. The truth is that every drug has side effects, even the so-called wonder drug aspirin.

As we are collectively vegging out in front of the TV, trying to recharge our batteries after a hard day at work, most of us do not even think twice when we watch a television commercial telling us how easy it is to take a pill that blocks heartburn, allowing you to eat the foods that you love.

What the marketing experts neglect to tell us, however, is the fact that the symptom of heartburn is your body's way of telling you that whatever you ate does not agree with your digestive system and may still cause long-term detrimental side effects, in addition to possible side effects from the heartburn medication that is designed to cover up outward symptoms.

None of us live in a perfect world, however, and no matter how hard we may try to create a healthy lifestyle, some factors, such as genetics and environmental factors are beyond our control. There are a multitude of instances where prescription drugs save lives and improve the health and longevity of the patient. In many cases, prescription or over-the-counter drugs are necessary, but far too many people use them for temporary relief of symptoms and conditions without considering the long-term consequences or attempting to do anything about the root cause of their health problems.

Considering the fact that stress is a leading cause of death in our modern world, it simply makes sense to focus your energy on prevention and reduction of the stress that you can control in your life. Instead of adding drug-induced side effects to the list of symptoms associated with stress-related conditions, try to pay attention to the warning signs and signals from your body's inborn, innate intelligence and take charge of the stress level in your life.

One good place to begin is by understanding the physiology of stress, which can help you deal more effectively with this widespread potential killer. Quick, shallow breathing, tense, knotted muscles (especially in the neck and back), and an increased heart rate are all signs that your body is under stress and feels threatened. Perhaps your jaw also tightens or you feel pressure in your chest or burning in your stomach.

When your body perceives a situation as being threatening, it responds with a rush of stress related chemicals, including adrenaline. When released in excessive amounts over time, adrenaline can upset your body's delicate biochemical balance. Prolonged, serious stress can actually deplete the adrenal glands. Another effect of stress is that more acid is secreted into the stomach, which can eventually lead to indigestion and other disturbances of the sensitive gastrointestinal system.

These responses are all part of your body's instinctive fight or flight reflex. This reflex comes in handy if you are being chased by a bear in the woods, but not if you are late for an important meeting and stuck in a frustrating bumper to bumper traffic jam. Unfortunately, when your body is under continuous, negative stress for prolonged periods of time, your pure energy level can be drained and depleted.

The rapid pace at which our complex world is changing can also cause you to develop an underlying sense of urgency and anxiety, often making normal, everyday situations feel like minor emergencies.

One of the powerful secrets to reducing the stress in your life is to learn to slow down internally and externally, in order to focus on connecting with the life force that is always there within you. This life force is the ultimate source of the powerful energy that travels throughout your body along the pathways of your autonomic nervous system, making it possible for your body to perform millions of intricate functions, far surpassing the capability of any manmade technology.

This awesome energy does not skip a beat as it pumps approximately two thousand gallons of blood through your heart every day and keeps a steady flow of air circulating through your lungs. The amazing thing is that your body does all this naturally and automatically, without your conscious awareness of all the minute details and complicated processes.

Unfortunately, there is no way to avoid stress totally. It is an inevitable part of life. How you choose to cope with stressful situations, however, plays a great role in the overall state of your health. Even when we cannot choose the outer conditions of our lives, we can still choose how we will respond to them.

Since the daily stress of life is often the primary obstacle that causes many people to take the wrong path or backtrack during the early portion of their Pure Life journey, I encourage you to take full advantage of the second helpful stepping stone, that your ancient Pura Vida guides carefully placed along the path only after slipping and falling many times themselves. If you look closely, you will find the second stepping stone partially hidden among the gnarled vines, sharp thorns, and barbs of the sometimes cruel concrete jungle.

Stepping Stone #2: *The second crucial stepping stone along your Pure Life path is to make a conscious effort to prevent and reduce the negative effects of stress in your daily life.*

Conquering the daily physical and emotional challenges of stress takes time and effort, but you will be much better equipped to handle the next unexpected stressful incident that comes your way after integrating the following recommendations into your daily lifestyle.

If you are over stimulated by stress, pay special attention to your consumption of caffeine. Practice what you learned from using the first stepping stone, listening to your innate intelligence. Your body usually lets you know when you have consumed too much caffeine. Increased feelings of anxiety, shakiness, insomnia, and even irregular heartbeats can all be warning signs from your body, telling you that the temporary energy boost that you may have received was not worth the long term, energy draining side effects of excessive caffeine consumption.

Eating a well balanced, nutritious diet that includes plenty of fresh, whole foods is also vital to maintaining consistent energy levels and efficiently preventing anxiety and reducing your stress level throughout your busy day. Conversely, skipping meals or eating junk food can leave you tired and with less energy to handle stressful situations.

Prolonged stress depletes the body's stores of protein, and may produce certain chemicals that lead to the production of cancer-causing free radicals. Stress can also deplete your body of vital nutrients, including cancer-fighting antioxidants.

These are just a few of the reasons why it is so important to make an effort to eat properly when you are under stress. Unfortunately, a healthy diet is usually one of the first things to go when people find themselves with too much to do each day, and not enough time to do it all in.

How often you eat and how you combine your meals is equally as important as how much you eat. By eating smaller, more frequent, light meals and healthy snacks throughout the day, you will provide your body with an ongoing, continuous source of energy and keep your blood sugar at a more consistent level.

In addition, anyone who exercises regularly knows what a powerful ally physical exertion and movement can be in counteracting stress. There is no feeling in the world quite like the natural high of exercise, because you are doing exactly what your brilliant body was designed to do. Since your body was made to be active, every part of it functions best when you keep moving on a regular basis.

Exercise connects you with the core source of your pure energy and makes you feel fully alive. Part of the scientific explanation for the euphoric feeling often associated with vigorous exercise is related to the release of pleasure-producing chemicals called endorphins. Endorphins are actually natural hormones that are released during some forms of strenuous exercise of long duration.

Although research has yet to establish whether or not there is a direct cause and effect relationship between elevated levels of endorphins and euphoric feelings during prolonged exercise, there is a definite association between the two factors.

Endorphin secretion has also been associated with increased pain tolerance, improved appetite control, and a reduction in anxiety, tension, and anger. Especially important to women is the implication of endorphins in the regulation of the female menstrual cycle. Recently, other factors such as alpha brain waves, neurotransmitters, and elevated body temperature have also been linked to the sense of well-being that often accompanies vigorous exercise.

As a specific response to stress, certain glands of the body produce stress hormones, which can build up and cause anxiety. Exercise can stimulate the release of natural substances that counteract the negative effects of these harmful stress hormones. I have always found this reaction a beautiful illustration of the body's natural ability to balance itself under the proper conditions.

I have been experiencing the positive physiological, psychological, and even spiritual benefits of regular exercise throughout my life, and can personally vouch for the stress reducing benefits of consistent exercise. In my experience, the sense of well-being and so-called exercise high occurs not only during exercise, but perhaps more importantly, continues to have a positive effect throughout the remainder of the day and sometimes into the next few days.

Like many of you, I have also found that consistent exercise dramatically increases the quality and amount of my own pure energy level, increases my confidence and stamina, and strengthens my immune system. Regular exercise can also help prevent insomnia, without subjecting your body to the negative side effects of sleeping pills.

People who are under stress often say that they simply do not have enough energy to exercise. What many of them do not realize, however, is that the exertion of energy in the right direction eventually creates more pure energy, and that by avoiding exercise, they may actually be increasing their stress level, rather than relieving it.

Once people begin to fully understand how closely related stress, exercise, and energy are, they often come to the realization that part of their stress and anxiety stems from the fact that they simply do not obtain a sufficient amount of physical activity and exercise.

When you are under stress, worrying and dwelling on negative thoughts only serves to intensify the situation. Instead of draining your valuable energy by thinking unproductive thoughts that only serve to attract like energy, engage in some sort of physical activity. Turn off the television, put on your headphones and running shoes and take the dog for a walk. Put on some peaceful music and get up and do a ten minute stretching routine, or go outside and play ball with the kids. If you have the time and opportunity, take a spinning class or hit a punching bag with boxing gloves.

Simply by moving your body, even if it is during a bad day swinging wildly on the golf course, or a routine morning cleaning house, you are supplying your brain with more oxygen. Keep in mind that increased oxygen to the brain results in increased mental function and powers of concentration.

Personally, whenever I find myself starting to worry or become anxious, I make a conscious effort to break the negative pattern by engaging in some form of exercise or physical activity. As soon as possible, I take a brisk walk or run, ride my bike, go inline skating, swim in the ocean, or work out.

I have had many of my most successful and creative brainstorms while participating in some form of physical exercise. In fact, many of the ideas for this book seemed to spring up out of nowhere while I was exercising. It is amazing how often the answers to your problems seem to be staring you in the face after a good, hard workout.

Avoiding excessive consumption of caffeine, eating properly, breathing deeply, and stretching and exercising regularly are just a few of the important tools you need for preventing and reducing the negative effects of stress in your daily life. In the following chapters, we will explore even more ways to avoid this common pitfall along your path of optimal health.

The way I see it, every day you wake up and have a new chance to be headed in either the right direction or the wrong direction. If you have not already begun implementing these stress prevention and reduction changes in your healthy life-style, start now. If you have already integrated these changes into your daily way of life, congratulations! You are definitely on the right track.

The Breath Of Life

Along with exercise and eating properly, there is something that you can begin doing at this very moment that will have an immediate effect on calming your nerves and reducing stress. It is the first thing that you did when you miraculously entered this world after living in a fluid filled environment for nine months, and you have not stopped since that time.

Breathing is such a natural, everyday activity, that its powerful benefits are often underestimated or ignored. By mastering diaphragmatic or deep belly breathing, you can significantly lower your heart rate and prevent or lessen feelings of anxiety and panic.

Breathing is a vital link between your conscious and subconscious mind. The circulation of air through your lungs is an automatic, involuntary action—you breathe whether you think about it or not. Breathing is unique, however, in that it is an involuntary action over which you can have conscious control.

The belief in the vital importance of focused deep breathing is deeply interwoven into the fabric of numerous religions and various cultures throughout the world. During our adventures in Costa Rica, Len and I witnessed a tradition involving breathing that we found very touching and spiritually meaningful.

One sunny afternoon, our humble friend Abeulo discovered a magnificent green bird that resembled a small toucan lying on the ground near our cabina. It appeared that the bird had flown into a window and was temporarily stunned. We were in a boisterous mood upon returning from a sublime hike in the cloudforest, when we encountered Abeulo gently holding the motionless bird.

Surprised to find him sitting quietly in the grass, we watched with awe as he patiently waited for the bird to stir, then reverently blew air around its large beak before releasing it into the crisp blue sky. As we watched the innocent, wildly beautiful creature fly away, Abeulo said something about breathing life back into the bird.

Despite the language barrier, we understood the deeper meaning behind his heartfelt gesture. During that magical moment, we all felt our spirits soar as the bird lifted itself free from the entanglements of our world and returned to the clean, fresh air high above us.

It is easy to take the simple act of breathing for granted when we are caught up in the sometimes turbulent flow of daily living. Only when we are in a situation where our oxygen flow is significantly restricted do we truly appreciate the crucial necessity of this amazing bodily function.

Stepping Stone #3: *For many reasons, practicing consistent deep diaphragmatic breathing is a vital component of your Pura Vida journey, and is the third helpful stepping stone along your own unique path.*

Thousands of years ago, the ancient seekers of truth in many cultures discovered something that we are only recently rediscovering in our modern society. By integrating deep breathing into our daily lifestyles, we are not only reducing stress and negative emotions, but also reinforcing the direct link between our conscious and subconscious minds, creating a more connected, balanced, and harmonious state of being. Practicing and utilizing deep breathing techniques increases your pure energy reserves and can create a sense of heightened awareness, clarity, and inner strength.

When under stress, most people have a tendency to hold their breath or breathe short, shallow breaths from the chest while tensing their muscles, especially the muscles of the jaw and neck. These actions significantly decrease the oxygen supply to the brain and consequently intensify feelings of anxiety or panic.

The next time you find yourself slipping into your usual way of dealing with a stressful situation, immediately stop and concentrate on your breathing. The most effective thing you can do to break the cycle of mishandling a stressful situation is to breathe deeply and continuously from your stomach.

Even though the average person breathes about twenty thousand times a day, many of us are still starved for oxygen because we do not breathe deeply enough. Since oxygen is necessary to produce pure energy, we end up feeling tired and stressed when we breathe too lightly. Lack of fresh air in our home and stagnant air in our work environments also results in a decreased level of oxygen supplied to the brain, making it difficult for us to think clearly.

If you find yourself sighing frequently—rapidly and sporadically inhaling and forcibly expelling a quick burst of air—it could be a sign that you are not breathing deeply enough throughout your busy day.

Most of us use only a small portion of our lungs for breathing, which allows stale air to build up in the unused portions. Fortunately, deep breathing and aerobic exercise help exchange this stale air for fresh air because these activities use more of the total lung space.

Oxygen is carried to your heart, brain, and the rest of your body by your blood. Breathing from the upper chest (also called shallow breathing) automatically limits the amount of oxygen that you take in. For your blood to carry a sufficient amount of oxygen to all of the different parts of your body, it must circulate faster when you do not breathe deeply enough. For this reason, shallow breathing puts a strain on the cardiovascular system and can contribute to high blood pressure.

Practicing deep diaphragmatic breathing is an essential component of expressing your Pure Life potential. Perhaps I believe in this practice so wholeheartedly because I was fortunate enough to have experienced the healing effects of deep breathing in the lush rainforests of Costa Rica. Square mile for square mile, more oxygen is produced in the dense vegetation of the world's rainforests than in any other place on earth.

All plants act as air purifiers, and give off oxygen in the air that we breathe. The interdependent cycle involving the exchange of carbon dioxide and oxygen by man, trees, and plants is a perfect example of how closely interrelated everything on this fragile planet truly is. As humans, we give off carbon dioxide, which trees need to flourish, when we breathe. In turn, trees give off oxygen, which we require for our survival. I believe that this healthy cycle of exchange between man and nature is one of the reasons that many people feel more energized when they spend time in a natural environment.

For this reason, you should purposely make an effort to expel as much of your residual volume of stale air as possible and replace it with fresh air when you find yourself deep in the woods or in some other natural setting where the air is fresh and clean.

I can recall several times in my life when I was walking in old growth areas, such as California's Muir Woods, that I experienced an almost surreal, heightened sense of awareness after practicing this method of breathing.

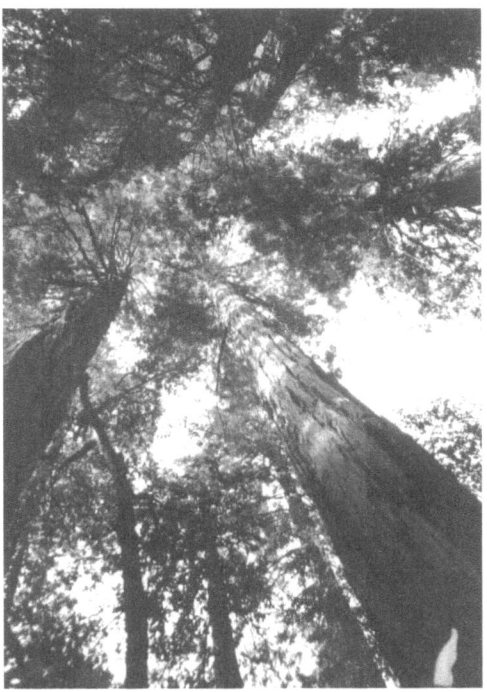

I attributed the sensation to the increased quality and amount of oxygen in the air. Although you will gain more positive benefits by practicing deep breathing outdoors, close to nature, it can be done anywhere and is simple to learn.

I believe so passionately in the importance of deep breathing that I have developed my own safe stretching method called Zoga, which incorporates the practice of deep abdominal breathing throughout. This daily stretching routine consists of a flowing series of safe and gentle stretches, starting with Breath of Life, the deep breathing, centering exercise described below. It is my favorite way of calming my busy mind and beginning my daily stretching practice.

You can learn more about the Zoga method of safe stretching by visiting www.pure-life.com and clicking on the Zoga link. Here you will find out more about the benefits of performing the gentle stretches that make up the Zoga routine. You will also find additional practical information and advice concerning stretching in Chapter 28 of this book.

If you performed only one exercise from the many integral exercises in the Zoga daily stretching routine, I would recommend the Breath of Life exercise as a way of centering your mind, reducing stress, and focusing on the connection between your mind and your body. To increase your understanding of exactly what should happen to your body as you practice correct deep breathing, please take a moment now to familiarize yourself with the simple Breath of Life exercise below.

First, pay attention to how you are breathing at this very moment. Are you breathing long, slow, deep breaths from your stomach, or short shallow breaths from your chest? Look at your stomach. Does it expand and contract as you breathe? With optimal deep abdominal breathing, your stomach should visibly expand as you inhale and contract as you exhale.

Now, stand in an upright position with your head up, shoulders back, and arms relaxed. Place your hands loosely around your waist with your fingers touching your lower rib cage and upper stomach.

Take a slow, deep breath in through your nose. Breathing in through your nose naturally filters the air, while breathing through your mouth does not. As you inhale, you should feel your rib cage and stomach noticeably expand under your fingertips. After your stomach has filled with air, your chest should expand slightly on the last part of the in-breath.

Now, slowly release the breath through your mouth, using your abdominal muscles to push your stomach in, gently forcing out the stale air that has built up in your lungs over time. You should be able to feel your abdominal muscles contracting under your fingers as you exhale.

When breathing correctly, you should be able to hear yourself slowly breathing in through your nose and out through your mouth. The deeper you inhale and exhale, the more you will be exchanging old stale air with fresh, new, energizing, oxygenated air.

Repeat this exercise as often as you wish being careful not to hyperventilate. Temporarily return to your normal pattern of breathing if you become dizzy or light headed while practicing this exercise. If you are a consistently shallow breather, it may take your body some time to adapt to this new way of exchanging air through your lungs.

Some people find it helpful to count as they practice deep diaphragmatic breathing. Personally, I have found that it is more important to listen to your body in order to establish an easy rhythm and span of time that is uniquely right for you. Although in this particular exercise, you are standing with your fingers on your ribcage and stomach, you can use the basic premise of this simple technique in all of your daily activities.

If you find yourself stuck in rush hour traffic or waiting in a long line, why not use the time to concentrate on improving your deep breathing skills? With repeated practice, your lung capacity will eventually grow, and you will be increasing the level of oxygen to your brain and all other parts of your body on a regular basis.

Once you have mastered deep, diaphragmatic breathing, it is extremely beneficial to integrate some form of meditation, which we will explore together in the next chapter, into your Pura Vida lifestyle. For now, however, take the time to practice this breathing technique, keeping in mind that deep breathing is a solid, practical stepping stone on your voyage, not simply some idealistic trend.

Almost everyone, at one time or another in their life, has longed to soar like Abuelo's wild bird, high above the chaos and confusion of our rapidly changing world. If you are feeling somewhat stunned and anxious about the challenges and obstacles of the concrete jungle, perhaps it is time to allow Mother Nature and your innate intelligence to breathe some life back into you.

Give yourself permission to slow down, smell the flowers, and take the time necessary to create a more peaceful, powerful, and energetic state of being by practicing deep breathing on a consistent basis. Not only will you be preventing and reducing stress, but you will also discover an internal state of harmony simply by doing what comes naturally—breathing the energizing breath of pure life!

Meditation

Meditation can be simply described as an active process of focusing the mind into a state of heightened awareness. By learning to be still and focused through meditation, you can reduce the negative effects of stress on your body, restore your pure energy level, and achieve a higher level of well-being. You will also experience more meaningful real moments when you take time to slow down and live fully in the present.

Many problems that are caused or aggravated by stress often improve with the practice of meditation. Meditation tends to lower or normalize blood pressure, pulse rate, and the levels of stress hormones in the blood.

High cholesterol and high blood pressure are often affected positively by daily meditation, as are anxiety, PMS, insomnia, and even infertility. If you suffer from chronic pain in the form of headaches or backaches, you may also find some relief by incorporating meditation into your daily lifestyle.

In addition to these valuable health benefits, I have personally found that I attain my practical, physical goals much more easily when I develop my mental muscles. In addition, I have found that regular practice of meditation can inspire creativity, as well as increase memory, intelligence, and the ability to concentrate.

One of the concepts that meditation has taught me personally is that if you want to change the outer circumstances of your life, it is necessary to focus on your inner life as well. When you focus your energy on obtaining inner peace, it is possible to create a quiet refuge where you can rise above the sometimes turbulent, complicated events of daily living.

When it feels as if the demands of the world are weighing heavily on their shoulders, spending time and energy on activities such as deep breathing and meditation may seem like a low priority to many people. Considering the enormous amount of time, energy, and hard earned money that Americans spend treating the symptoms of stress related conditions, however, our society would benefit tremendously by making these activities a much higher priority.

There are numerous meditation techniques that can be explored through books, classes, and qualified individuals, to help you find the one that works best for you. Fortunately, it is not necessary to wear brightly colored robes, while sitting cross-legged, burning incense, and chanting to experience the positive benefits of meditation. What is really important is that you learn to quiet your mind in your own uniquely personal way and use the wisdom gained from the first stepping stone by listening closely to your innate intelligence.

There are many different forms of meditation, from transcendental meditation, which involves internally reciting a mantra or holy sound, to mindful exercises such as *qi gong*, in which practitioners perform graceful movements while meditating on the flow of *chi* (life force) throughout their bodies. Some people consider taking a long, hot bath, going for a quiet walk on the beach, or performing repetitive tasks such as knitting or weeding their garden a form of meditation.

For many people, including myself, a process called progressive relaxation induces the relaxation response, which helps counteract the negative effects of the body's fight or flight response to stress. For me, progressive relaxation usually begins with some creative visualization, as discussed earlier.

Once I have visualized my oasis of *tranquilo*, and concentrated my focus on slowing down and utilizing proper deep breathing techniques, I continue the process of progressive relaxation. This technique is often recommended by mental health professionals to help relieve muscle tension and produce a sharpened state of awareness and mental clarity.

While sitting comfortably in a quiet, safe place with your eyes closed, you can begin the process by contracting and relaxing each muscle group of the body, beginning at the top, with the face and neck. Then, progressively tense, hold for a few seconds, and relax the muscles of your upper chest, shoulders, arms, abdomen, hips, buttocks, thighs, knees, and calves—all the way down to your feet.

Practice what you have learned by utilizing the second stepping stone, breathing deeply from your stomach throughout the process, while continuing to visualize your tranquil oasis. You may repeat this procedure two or three times if you wish.

After effectively releasing muscle tension through this process, I usually move on to a still, quiet focusing of my mind. For many people, this is the most difficult aspect of meditation—sitting still for an extended period of time, quieting and relinquishing busy thoughts.

With discipline and practice, however, your mind will eventually calm down. As thoughts continue to drift into your mind, it helps to think of them as bubbles floating upward and out of sight, leaving behind a clean, uncluttered slate of quiet and calmness.

Although you may not be consciously aware of it, your subconscious often uses this time to solve problems or resolve conflicts that may be confronting you, and also to stimulate creative inspiration. It is crucial to concentrate on your breathing throughout the experience of meditation in order to experience maximum benefits.

Many people find it helpful to sit it a yoga position with their legs crossed and their back straight while meditating. While this traditional position helps facilitate nerve flow, over time it can stress the knee joints in certain individuals. My best advice is to find a comfortable position that works for you on a long-term basis. I have found that sitting comfortably in a chair or even lying face up on a very thick cushioned yoga mat can help put me in a meditative state.

Simply lying flat on your back and letting your body become heavy also induces a calm and relaxed state for most people. An extremely relaxing yoga pose known as *Savasana* is a tried and true relaxation tool that has stood the test of time. To perform this simple exercise, lie on your back with your arms to your sides. Rotate your legs in and out, and then let them fall gently out to the sides.

Let your arms fall alongside your body, slightly separated from the body, palms facing upwards. Rotate the spine by turning your head from side to side to center it. Then start stretching yourself out, as though someone is pulling your head away from your feet, your shoulders down and away from your neck, your legs down and away from your pelvis.

Breathe deeply and slowly from your abdomen. Hold the pose for several minutes. Make your mind still and concentrate on your breath. After doing the pose, bend your knees. Using your legs, push yourself onto one side and then push yourself into a sitting position. Not only does this exercise calm the body and nervous system, but it also helps decompress and traction out the spine and the body's core.

When you take time on a regular basis to nurture your soul and calm your mind and body through the practice of meditation, you will ultimately experience a deep, powerful sense of peace, a fresh perspective, and new, vital, pure energy.

Another crucial component of the Pura Vida lifestyle that is often overlooked in our busy world is the body's need for high quality sleep. During sleep, your body restores its energy level, heals, and transforms itself. If you have ever suffered from the physical and emotional effects of sleep deprivation, you know from personal experience that lack of sleep directly affects every other aspect of your life. Insomnia, like so many other conditions and symptoms, is often a warning sign from your body, telling you that something is out of balance in your lifestyle.

The amount and quality of the sleep that you obtain each night is determined by many factors—yet another example of how everything in your life is interrelated. Your stress level, the amount of exercise you obtain, and even your nutrient and water consumption all enter into the equation.

In the following chapters, I will answer some specific questions that you may have concerning proper sleeping positions and the use of pillows. I will also offer some practical, everyday advice that will help you create a healthier lifestyle and, in so doing, achieve a higher state of physical, mental, and spiritual well-being.

At this point in your journey, however, you can continue to establish a solid, healthy foundation by assimilating techniques such as deep breathing, creative visualization, meditation, and progressive relaxation into your daily lifestyle.

Integrating practices such as these into your daily routine can have a dramatic impact on your energy level and contribute not only to spiritual growth and renewal but also to a more balanced and harmonious physical state. We can all benefit by taking time to nourish our souls, quiet the extraneous noise from the outside world, and listen to that still, small voice within.

Your body's inborn intelligence has many of the answers to the questions you may be asking. Often, all you have to do is stop and listen to what your remarkable, intelligent body is trying to tell you.

Positive Body Image

Your body truly is your temple, but the sad reality is, many people take better care of their automobiles than their own bodies. Very few of us treat our bodies with the full respect that they deserve.

Stepping Stone # 4: *Respecting and loving your body exactly as it is at this moment is the fourth stepping stone on your Pura Vida journey.*
The ancient Pura Vida trailblazers placed this simple stepping stone thousands of years ago without much trouble. They instinctively listened to their body's innate intelligence, living simply, and in a peaceful and harmonious state of coexistence with their environment.

After achieving new heights along the Pura Vida path by using this stepping stone, respecting and honoring your physical body and appreciating all of the amazing things that it does for you, you may also come to fully appreciate some of the more detailed, intricate workings of your miraculous body.

You appreciate that, as you are reading this book, your immune system is valiantly fighting off harmful bacteria and viruses, and your kidneys are delicately filtering out toxins. You respect your body for having the stamina and endurance to see you through hard times and still get up out of bed and go to work day after day.

When you truly love and respect your body, inside and out, you will find that it is easier to maintain your own uniquely individual, ideal healthy body shape and size. You will want to stay in shape and eat properly because of the way that taking care of yourself makes you feel—more alive and energetic, better prepared for life's many challenges. You will avoid unhealthy extremes and ignore the media's unattainable ideals of steroid-pumped young men, and thin, teenage models who sometimes starve themselves and abuse their bodies.

As I witnessed in my practice and by working out in gyms most of my adult life, the number of teenagers and adults who endanger their lives by using anabolic steroids for body building purposes is truly alarming. Not only can steroid use cause psychotic behavior, but it can also have dangerous, irreversible side effects on the cardiovascular system, liver, and reproductive organs.

I find it incomprehensible that a person would risk his or her life for the temporary appearance of abnormally large muscles and unattractive bulging veins. Steroid use seems especially ridiculous when you consider that almost everyone can attain a firm, healthy looking physique that is much more attractive to the average person, naturally, without the health threatening side effects of drugs.

Ours is a very body conscious society, but for all of the wrong reasons. Having a strong body with some muscular definition is important, but not simply because you want to look good in your jeans. Your physical appearance can be an outward indicator of how well you are treating your inner body. Excessively weak, flabby muscles and an abnormal amount of excess bodyfat are not merely unattractive, cosmetic problems. They are a warning sign, a symptom that something is out of balance in your physical body or your overall lifestyle.

The same inactive lifestyle that causes your muscles to become weak is also a contributing factor in conditions such as osteoporosis and cardiovascular disease. The same fatty substances that lodge in and block arterial walls, causing heart disease, contribute to the formation of love handles and saddlebags, as well.

Throughout history, the sages of most societies have practiced the crucial principle of Pure Energy Balance. This principle is a core component of the Pura Vida Philosophy and therefore is represented by a major stepping stone—the fifth along your path thus far.

This solid stone is lodged firmly above the slippery roots and organic, decaying leaves of a giant banyan tree that grows and thrives directly in relation to the amount of sunlight, nutrients, water, and carbon dioxide it receives.

Stepping Stone #5: *Integrate the Pure Energy Balance Principle into all aspects of your daily lifestyle.*

For example, on a nutritional level, Pure Energy Balance is the healthy balance between your intake of food (your energy input) and your exertion of physical energy (your energy output). If you do not take in sufficient energy in the form of calories and nutrients from your diet, it simply stands to reason that you will not have enough energy to lead an active, healthy lifestyle. Likewise, if you take in poor quality energy, your energy output will be poor. If you consume too much energy in the form of calories, you will eventually have excess stored body fat.

On another level, the principle of energy balance also includes absorbing positive energy from healthy relationships, productive, creative, and joyful experiences, and other aspects of living a healthy lifestyle.

Your energy output is directly related to the amount and quality of energy that you take in from various sources. For example, we have all been around somewhat toxic people who literally drain our energy. I often think of those people as energy vampires. Conversely, each of us has spent time with energizing people or had positive experiences with others that made us feel literally full of life for extended periods of time afterward.

On a nutritional level, you are utilizing the Energy Balance stepping stone when you make it a high priority to take care of your body and establish the correct balance between eating the proper amounts and types of food, and obtaining your ideal amount of exercise and activity. In doing so, you will naturally discover the realistic, positive body image that is healthy for you.

Do not be overly concerned if this healthy weight does not match the magic number recommended by generalized weight and bodyfat percentage charts. What matters most is that you treat your body with respect, and that you maintain a consistently balanced, healthy lifestyle.

In this world of seductive, subliminal advertising and psychologically manipulative money making schemes, it is all too easy to become trapped in the never ending cycle of getting excited about a new quick weight loss program or product only to find out later that it was more hype than help.

One of the many problems with this frustrating cycle is that you spend valuable time and energy that could have been used to permanently change your lifestyle and steadily progress on a common sense course on the road to health. Eventually, you wind up losing ground when you have to backtrack on a path that initially looked promising, but in actuality led to a dead end or circled back around to the starting point.

I have found that my health related progress is much more rapid when I think for myself and consciously make the decision not to be influenced by the latest hype and nonsense surrounding magic bullet products, diets, or programs.

Do not allow yourself to become caught up in the swinging pendulum of extremes in life. If you have ever practically starved yourself to lose weight, only to gain more pounds back after a subsequent period of unrestricted, unhealthy eating, or if you have ever been completely sidelined by an injury caused by over exercising, you have already experienced the futility of going to extremes in your daily lifestyle.

The next time some self-proclaimed fitness expert or miracle diet promoter shouts obnoxiously at you from your television, do not simply try to block it out. Turn off the television or simply change the channel.

Instead, learn from your own life experiences and trust your body's innate intelligence to provide the answers and guidance that you are seeking. Trust your own intuition. It will speak to you in a number of ways, whether it is a gut feeling, a bodily sensation, or simply a strong sense of right or wrong.

Your mind and body coexist in a flowing yin-yang type relationship. Your conscious and subconscious thoughts constantly affect the physical state of your body. Conversely, the signals from your body, including physical pain, pleasure, and discomfort, have a direct effect on your mind and emotional state. Therefore, an imbalance in one naturally creates an imbalance in the other.

Since true health and healing cannot be achieved unless there is a healthy balance between the Pure Life Triune of mind, body, and spirit, it is crucial for all of us to spend time engaging in activities, such as exercise, meditation, and deep breathing, that merge physical and mental energies simultaneously. Those who do achieve this state of holistic fusion usually find that respecting and loving their physical body, just as it is, is a natural result of spending time strengthening the Pure Life Triune connection.

Your body is a miraculous, hard working masterpiece that should be loved, honored, and treated with respect. It is much more than simply a machine or the vehicle that carries you along on your journey through life.

My experience as a health care provider to thousands of patients has offered me numerous opportunities to gain a deeper appreciation and respect for the human body. Several experiences were beyond my everyday realm of belief and true testaments to the healing power within us all.

My most dramatic experience involved a young patient's permanently contracted finger straightening out after several gentle adjustments to his neck region. Other healing experiences were not quite as dramatic but just as meaningful on other levels.

One of my favorite patients was the victim of a stroke and basically bedridden for the last twelve years. In working with her, I was given the lasting gift of appreciation for the simple act of walking, and being able to go wherever I want whenever I want. Seeing the longing in her eyes as she shared a dream from the night before about walking in the rain and feeling the mud between her toes moved me in a way that I will never forget.

Although educating others has always been a high priority for me, I have often thought that my patients have collectively taught me more than I have them over the years. In addition, they have inspired me and reminded me that we are all bigger than our bodies and much more than what the eye can see.

Your remarkable body makes it possible for you to move, think, work, play, live, laugh, and love. Can you imagine how much more fully each of us would enjoy all of these actions if we treated our body like the temple that it truly is?

Strong, Confident, Healthy Posture

Your self-image, and the way others view you, are directly affected by your body posture. We have all observed people who seem to draw attention and attract positive energy to themselves, simply because of the confident, self-assured way that they carry themselves through a room, or briskly stride down a crowded street.

Conversely, poor posture is very often related to poor self-image. You have probably noticed that many people with slumped posture have a tendency to look helpless, weak, and tired. Some people seem to literally carry the weight of the world on their shoulders.

There are many causes of poor posture, including structural and biomechanical problems that should be treated by a qualified professional. Some of the possible negative effects of poor posture are muscular pain, headaches, neck and back pain, fatigue, reduced lung capacity, and reduced levels of blood and oxygen supplied to the brain.

Since some spinal conditions can only be detected by x-rays or by thorough physical examination, I personally believe that it is a good idea to consult a qualified Doctor of Chiropractic for a spinal checkup, even if you are not currently experiencing pain or symptoms.

As far back as 1250 BC, the ancient Greeks were looking to the spine as a cause of dis-ease in the human body. The nerves exiting the spinal cord through the openings of the spinal column directly supply the pure energy that regulates and controls every system of your body. A healthy spine positively affects the free flow of pure energy throughout all the systems of your body, including the digestive, reproductive, respiratory, and immune systems.

As a chiropractor who has treated thousands of patients over the years, I have personally witnessed the phenomenal healing and energizing power of the human nervous system on a daily basis. Consequently, I truly believe that maintaining a strong, healthy, properly aligned spinal column is essential to achieving overall health and optimal well being in your daily life. A healthy spine is the strong foundation of a healthy body.

Strengthening the muscles of the back increases the stability of the spinal column and can help prevent serious problems caused by musculoskeletal imbalance. By balancing the strength in the front and the back of your body, you will have less chance of injury in your daily activities.

Usually, the most under exercised muscles in the body are in the back. Building up some muscles, while ignoring others, may pull your body out of balance. For example, if you develop strong chest and abdominal muscles without working on strengthening your back, you will eventually start to slump over. Strengthening the hamstring and core abdominal muscles also helps stabilize the spinal column, due to the connection of these muscles to the pelvis.

Exercising both sides of your body evenly can prevent imbalance of muscle strength on either side of the spine. Muscular imbalance can be a result of overuse of the muscles on one side, and under use on the other and can eventually lead to structural imbalance of the bones and joints.

In my opinion, a daily routine of stretching is one of the most important tools that you have in preventing pain, decreasing spasm, reducing stress and improving posture. A regular program of safe stretching can decrease muscular imbalance and help elongate the muscles of the spine and lower back. Fortunately, by performing the flowing series of stretches in the safe and gentle Zoga routine, you can dramatically improve your posture and increase everyday range of motion and flexibility.

Musculoskeletal imbalance can also be caused or aggravated by the type of work that you do, by unilateral sports such as tennis or golf, or by always favoring one side when you carry a briefcase, handbag, child, or other heavy object. Whenever possible, change sides or positions to prevent muscular imbalance and subsequent structural imbalance. Most of us favor one side or the other for certain activities in our daily lives without being consciously aware of our patterns.

I have seen hundreds of cases where an individual slouched because they were insecure or perceived themselves as being too tall for so many years that their posture was permanently altered as a result. Another example of a repetitive physical activity that negatively affects the musculoskeletal and nervous system over the years involves the cervical (neck) portion of the spinal column.

Any activity that requires you to look down for long periods, especially reading, computer use, and deskwork, can produce a chronic forward head position. Eventually, this repetitive strain can lead to a decrease of the normal C-shaped curve in the neck, which makes it difficult for the neck to support the heavy weight of the head.

Biomechanically speaking, the normal C-shaped curve in your neck makes it stronger, and with a decrease of that natural curve (which is sometimes the case after whiplash type injuries and ligament damage caused by trauma), the neck loses some of its weight-bearing strength. In chapter 36, I will discuss several practical ways to prevent and reduce spinal related pain and stiffness.

Fortunately, one of the most effective ways to improve your posture is simply to become more aware of it. Seeing yourself as others see you is often the first step to making improvements in your posture. I recommend evaluating your body in a full-length mirror from the side view—a position in which you rarely see yourself—viewing your posture while using a hand held mirror. You may even want to have a friend take a picture of you from the side, standing as you normally stand.

With correct posture, when viewed from the side, your ears are balanced directly above the arches of your feet, and your head is only slightly forward of the neck, shoulder blades, and lower back. A plumb line dropped from overhead should pass through the ear, shoulder, hip, knee, and ankle. Also assess your posture from the front view. Ideally, both of your hips, shoulders, and ears should be level. Your head should not tilt to one side or the other.

To help you become more aware of your posture, try the following exercise while standing in front of a mirror. Imagine two gentle hands on either side of your head pulling you upright, and a light helpful hand at your back pushing your shoulder blades together.

Think tall, lengthen your neck, and let your head move upward, with the chin slightly in. Breathe deeply from your stomach, pushing out your chest. Concentrate on lengthening your spine, still imagining the top of your head reaching toward the ceiling. Keep your stomach in and buttocks tucked. Slightly bend your knees without locking them, since locking your knees puts unnecessary stress on your lower back.

Now, visualize yourself walking with a certain Pure Life presence, a way of carrying your body that projects self-confidence and inner strength. Picture yourself with regal posture; head held high, shoulders back, feeling tall, proud, and self-assured.

Take a deep abdominal breath and imagine yourself on top of the sunlit peak that you visualized earlier on your allegorical journey, reaching your arms toward the sky, radiating pure life, pure energy, and pure health. With continued practice you will start looking and feeling like the self-confident person that you have always known you are.

I have always loved the old saying "To be, act as if." When you assume the body posture of a strong, energetic, and confident person, walking with a spring in your step and a smile on your face, you will find that the physiological changes also positively affect your mind and soul, lifting your spirits and sometimes even changing your whole outlook on life.

Once you have evolved to the point of truly loving your body by utilizing the fourth stepping stone, you will discover that it is easier to make time and energy to do whatever needs to be done. You may even want to explore different techniques for improving posture and spinal health including: Chiropractic, Yoga, Dance, Martial Arts, and various types of Bodywork Therapy, such as Pilates, Assisted Stretching, and different forms of Massage Therapy, such as Rolfing and Cranio Sacral work. Some of the most dramatic personal and physical changes that I have observed in the past few years have been the result of a combination of two or more of these types of methods.

Toward the end of this book, I will offer you further practical advice on more ways to improve your posture, strengthen your back, and prevent spinal and musculoskeletal injuries.

Taking some time to pay attention to your posture and take care of your spine is an integral component of achieving optimal health and expressing your pure life energy. Remember, it is how you carry yourself that counts. Think strong, energetic, and confident!

The Truth About Excess Bodyfat

Once you begin integrating all of the different aspects of your Pura Vida lifestyle with the aid of the various stepping stones, you will find that you are paying more attention to the warning signs that your body constantly offers you.

An abnormal amount of excess bodyfat is one of those signs or indicators. It is usually a signal telling you that you are taking in more food than your body needs to function, or that you are not obtaining sufficient exercise and physical activity in your daily lifestyle.

Other factors, such as heredity and metabolism also contribute to your physique. Recent evidence suggests that genes and heredity play a more important role in clinical obesity than previously believed. Although it is often hard to draw the line between obesity and being extremely overweight, both conditions can have an adverse effect on the quality of your life and your overall health and happiness.

Obesity can contribute to potentially life threatening heart, kidney, and circulatory diseases, not to mention diabetes and hormonal disturbances. Deaths due to cancers of the uterus, gallbladder, kidney, stomach, colon, breast, and other organs, have also been associated with obesity.

For some people, being even moderately overweight can have very real psychological consequences. Even if the excess weight is not life threatening, it can have a negative effect on all aspects of a person's life, from their personal and professional relationships, to the way they feel about themselves while walking across the street or trying on clothes.

It is a physiological fact of life that women naturally have more bodyfat than men. For most women, reducing the stubborn dimples and bulges on the hips and thighs is a unique, ongoing challenge. For this reason, I have included a helpful section regarding this matter specifically for women toward the end of this book. Men will benefit from reading this chapter, as well.

Women may naturally have more bodyfat than men but, unfortunately, for men, the consequences of being overweight can be especially life threatening. Research suggests that the risk of death from heart disease for men who are just 20% overweight is two and one-half times that for those whose weight is ideal.

Work related stress, improper diet, and insufficient exercise and activity are just a few of the factors that make staying at a healthy weight particularly challenging for both sexes in today's high tech world.

There is quite a contrast between the strenuous physical labor performed by our forefathers, and today's increasingly high stress and low physical activity office jobs. Our modern occupations are often a contributing factor to the alarming number of deaths resulting from heart attacks at frighteningly young ages.

The accumulation of large amounts of excess bodyfat resulting from inactivity and improper nutrition takes time. The situation does not develop overnight, and will not go away in a few weeks, despite what many so-called diet experts would like us to believe.

You can, however, noticeably reduce your fat stores much quicker and with a lot less frustration, if you know the facts. Here are some physiological facts that will help define your belief system as it relates to weight gain.

Excess bodyfat is basically stored energy. Dietary excesses, whether in the form of fats, carbohydrates, or protein, all eventually turn to bodyfat if they are not needed by the body as a source of energy.

Energy is stored by the body as fat in adipose tissue, which is a distinct type of connective tissue. When other sources of energy, such as glucose (blood sugar) are depleted, the body draws on fat stores for its needs.

Adipose tissue increases in two ways. Existing fat cells can grow by filling up with more fat, or the total number of fat cells can increase. As the original fat cells are filled to capacity, new ones are created.

I find it very interesting to note that when an overweight adult reduces body size, there is a decrease in fat cell size, but no change in total fat cell number. In other words, fat cells can shrink in size, but once new fat cells are created, they are there to stay.

The reason that most women gain weight more easily than men is related to the historical evolution of fat storage mechanisms as protection against starvation in periods of famine. In general, a man's body contains enough fat to protect itself for a few months. A woman's body, on the other hand, is designed to store enough fat to protect her and her unborn child for the length of a full term pregnancy.

The total amount of bodyfat in an individual's body is found in two storage sites, or depots. The first depot, essential fat, is required for normal physiological functioning. Essential fat is stored in major organs such as the heart, lungs, and liver. It is also stored in muscles, the marrow of bones, and in tissues of the central nervous system.

The other major fat depot, storage fat, consists of fat that accumulates in adipose tissue. People who strive to maintain an extremely low body fat content should be aware of a very important fact: one of the functions of storage fat is to protect the internal organs from trauma, such as car accidents and falls. As someone who has worked with hundreds of auto accident victims (both in the physical therapy department of a hospital and also in private chiropractic practice) I have come to appreciate the value of a little padding around the joints and bones for protective purposes.

Storage fat also includes the larger subcutaneous fat volume found beneath the skin surface. Subcutaneous fat (sub means under, cutaneous refers to the skin) is the sometimes visible storage fat found directly under the skin and on top of the muscles in the subcutaneous layer.

Your skin is composed of three layers: epidermis, dermis, and subcutaneous fatty tissue, which is actually the deepest layer of the skin. This tissue is made of a mesh-like network of connective tissue, fat cells, and blood vessels.

The subcutaneous fatty tissue layer stores energy in the form of fat, insulates your body from the cold, and binds the skin to underlying structures. Stored subcutaneous fat is deposited mainly around the hips, thighs, and abdomen.

Please note that in writing about reducing excess bodyfat throughout this book, I am referring to reducing excess stored subcutaneous fat. I am not referring to reducing the healthy amount of fat that is necessary for normal body functioning.

Also, please note that there is a major difference between losing bodyfat and losing weight. The term weight refers specifically to overall bodyweight, which includes bones, organs, skin, fluid, muscle, and fat. For this reason, fad diets that promise that you will be watching numbers rapidly drop on the scales are usually dangerous. Bodyfat is not the only thing that you lose on these diets. When you lose weight at an unhealthy rapid rate, you may also be losing vital muscle, water, protein, and glycogen, which your body needs in precisely the right amounts to function efficiently.

It is also imperative to understand that muscle and fat are two distinct types of tissue. You cannot burn fat and turn it into muscle. Conversely, unused muscle does not simply turn into fat.

When you begin or accelerate a strength training program, your existing muscles become larger in response to the amount of resistance placed on them. When you perform a sufficient amount of aerobic exercise, your body burns fat by using your existing fat stores as a source of fuel. Here is a little known fact that I discovered years ago in a physiology textbook that everyone should be aware of. It is one of my favorite little nuggets of truth and has helped me tremendously in my own exercise and fitness routine.

Many people spend fifteen or twenty minutes on the treadmill or stationary bike and mistakenly assume that they are burning fat the entire time. The process of burning fat as a fuel is a little more complicated than is commonly believed, however.

Let's say you are pedaling away on a recumbent bike trying to burn bodyfat. At the beginning stage of an aerobic exercise session such as this, your primary source of energy is from carbohydrates, which are stored as glycogen in the muscles.

For the next twenty minutes or so as you continue exercising, your glycogen stores supply only about half of your energy requirements, with the other half being provided by the breakdown of fat from the subcutaneous level.

The longer you exercise past this point, the more your glycogen stores are reduced, and a higher percentage of energy is supplied by the metabolism of fat. Even though the potential energy from stored fat is almost unlimited, you will eventually hit the wall or be too tired to continue if the glycogen stores in the liver and muscles becomes severely lowered.

To put it simply: In the warm up phase of aerobic exercise, you use mostly glycogen from carbohydrates. The longer you continue exercising, the more you will burn fat as a source of fuel. I call this principle the Twenty Minute Rule because only after about twenty minutes does your body start to use fat as its primary energy source. Consequently, to begin truly burning from your fat stores, you may need to participate in cardiovascular activities and exercises a little longer than you are accustomed to.

There is another factor that you should be aware of if you are trying to reduce excess bodyfat. Regular aerobic exercise actually changes your body's biochemistry so that you will burn fat more efficiently. This is largely due to the increase in fat burning enzymes. To stimulate this increase in fat burning enzymes, a minimum of twelve minutes of continuous, uninterrupted exercise is necessary.

Quite honestly, if you are extremely overweight, twenty minutes or a half-hour of exercising once or twice a week is not likely to dramatically melt off the fat. I recommend gradually working your way up to forty minutes of aerobic exercise for a minimum of three or four times a week if your primary goal is to lose significant amounts of excess bodyfat.

The key word here is *gradually*. Once again, it is crucial to listen carefully to your body and steadily build a healthy momentum that is uniquely right for you and in line with your goals and physical condition.

The awesome advantage of lengthier aerobic sessions is that they increase your metabolism long after you stop sweating, in some cases for up to six or seven hours. I have found that I often have a second wind somewhere after the half hour point and that the longer I exercise past that point, the greater the fat burning results.

While exercise can speed up your metabolism, the only way it can do so is if you supply your body with enough calories to support your extra energy requirements. It is both dangerous and unhealthy to take in insufficient calories and exercise excessively.

If you frequently sustain overuse injuries and find yourself consistently exhausted rather than energized after exercising, you are probably pushing your body past its healthy limits and may be doing more harm than good. Take care of and respect your body. It is your true home and must last you a lifetime.

If you weigh yourself frequently, please keep the following facts in mind. Muscle really does weigh more than fat—approximately two and one-half times more. The more muscle mass you have, the faster your metabolism is. Weight charts are only generalized guidelines and do not take into account factors such as your skeletal structure or the amount of muscle tissue that you have.

Also keep in mind that it is perfectly normal and healthy to have some visible body fat. Like every other component of your amazing body, fat has a necessary purpose and function and is there for a reason. Truly loving and respecting your body exactly as it is at this moment becomes much easier when you accept this simple fact.

It is much easier to keep your body fat at a level that is healthy for you when you listen to your body and consistently make the right choices rather than starve yourself, exercise excessively, or allow yourself to be caught up in an unhealthy cycle of weight loss and gain.

Only you know at what weight you feel most comfortable, healthy, and energetic. Do not waste valuable time and energy worrying about how much you weigh. Instead, concentrate on how physically fit and truly healthy you are—inside and out!

Pure H₂O

At one point in our Costa Rican adventures, Len and I spent about a week on the beautiful shores of Montezuma, a remote jungle town with limited access to quality drinking water. There was literally water, water everywhere with powerful waterfalls plunging into the ocean, but at that time, not a lot to drink that we could trust.

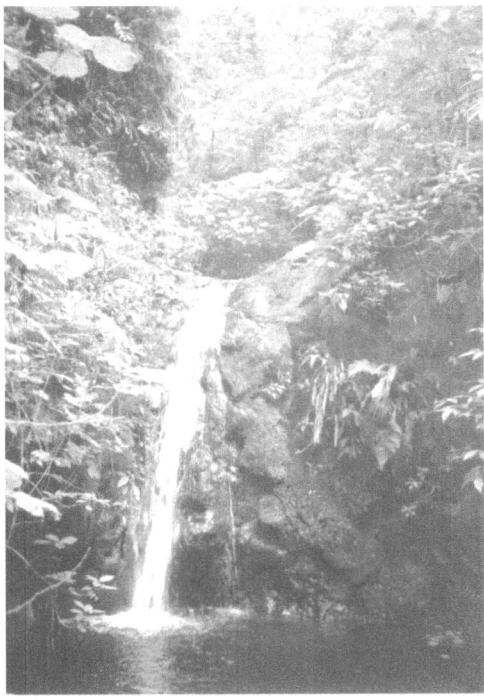

Luckily, we didn't suffer from Montezuma's revenge, but, as individuals whose bodies are accustomed to constantly drinking pure water throughout our normal day, we could immediately feel the negative effects of lowered levels of H20 on our health and overall energy level.

Someone once said that the best way to make a person appreciate what they have is to take it away from them, and then to give it back. We had always taken clean, pure, drinking water for granted and fully appreciated it only when we temporarily had this luxury taken away from us.

This experience taught me a valuable lesson that may very well be the same lesson that motivated the early Pura Vida trail blazers to place a wide, solid stepping stone in the middle of a steady, gushing stream running across the Pure Life path.

Stepping Stone #6: _Drinking plenty of pure water is the sixth helpful stepping stone in achieving the healthy lifestyle you deserve._

Water truly is the single most important nutrient that you can consume. Depending on the reference that you read, anywhere from 40–60% of an individual's body weight is water. Differences in total body water can vary greatly from person to person depending on body composition. This is largely due to the fact that water makes up 65–75 % of the weight of muscle and less than 25 % of the weight of fat. In other words, there is considerably more water content in muscles than there is in fat.

One of the reasons it is essential that you drink a minimum of eight glasses of water each day is that your body needs at least that much to replace what it loses daily. Fortunately, eating fruits and vegetables with high water content can help you meet some of your body's water requirements.

All of the major systems of your body need water to function properly, but very few of us drink enough H20. Your skin, the largest organ of the body, loses water every day through perspiration. Your lungs alone need about two glasses of water daily to work properly. Your small intestines and kidneys use large quantities of water for proper elimination as well.

Unfortunately, our bodies were not made to handle the thousands of preservatives, additives, and chemicals in the processed foods that make up so much of the average person's diet today. Since your body has no physiological need for these things, it processes and either disposes of or stores these and other impurities that we take in as toxins. Water helps flush toxins out of the body through the natural processes of elimination. In addition, waste products leave the body through the water in urine and feces.

Dietary toxins can build up over time if they are not excreted by the body. Not only does this put a strain on the kidneys and other organs of elimination, but it can also interfere with the delicate balance and flow of fluids in the tissues of the body.

The cells of your body are constantly bathed in fluid, and a proper flow of fluids into and out of the cells is necessary for optimal health. When this flow of fluids is disrupted, the internal cellular environment can become stagnant and unhealthy, resulting in a negative effect on your overall health.

Your lymphatic system disposes of your body's metabolic waste. In essence, it is your body's cleansing mechanism. Lymphatic fluid surrounds the cells and takes excess fluids and waste from the cells to the lymph nodes, where the fluid is filtered and cleaned. Sufficient amounts of water are necessary for your lymphatic system to work properly.

A popular misconception about water is that drinking large amounts causes bloating or puffiness, or causes you to retain weight. On the contrary, not drinking enough water can actually slow down fat loss. Often, it is actually excess sodium that causes fluid retention.

The common practice of taking diuretics for weight loss can be extremely dangerous because these products move some of the water that the body needs out of the system, which can slow down the elimination of waste products and toxins. Muscular cramps, loss of important minerals, and irregular heart rhythm are just a few of the dangerous side effects of diuretic abuse.

Try to keep track of how much water you drink. I highly recommend that you drink a minimum of eight, eight-ounce glasses of pure water every day, which is only half a gallon. Since drinking large amounts of water while eating can dilute the digestive enzymes, it is better to drink most of your water between meals rather than with them.

Len and I have designated cups and glasses at home that we use only for water, and we rarely leave the house without taking a water bottle with us. We like using heavy, dishwasher proof plastic water bottles with a small mouth and screw on lid, available wherever you find camping gear, for our away from home water needs. To remind yourself to drink more water, I recommend keeping a glass or bottle of water beside you at home, on your nightstand, on your desk at work, and especially during exercise.

It is important to note that as activity increases, so do your body's fluid needs. An hour before a strenuous cardiovascular workout, I always try to drink one glass of water, then drink another glass fifteen minutes later. During my workout, I drink small amounts every twenty minutes or so. Afterwards, I try to drink a sufficient amount of water to replace the fluids that were lost.

You cannot use thirst as an accurate indicator of how much water to drink, especially if you are very active or live in a hot climate. If you wait until your brain sends the signal that you are thirsty, often the fluid level in your body is already too low, and you risk dehydration.

Drinking alcoholic beverages stimulates water loss and can have a dehydrating effect on the body. Caffeine can also have a dehydrating effect because caffeine speeds up the kidneys' function, causing the body to process water more rapidly.

Imagine yourself in the following scenario along your everyday journey through life: You are paying for gas inside a convenience store. It is brutally hot outside and you are thirsty, so you find yourself standing in front of the glass doors of the refrigerator case, trying to decide what to drink. Whether you are aware of it or not, your subconscious mind is being bombarded with the cumulative result of billions of dollars worth of advertising and subliminal visual stimuli as you try to make your decision.

In a matter of seconds, many thoughts go through your mind. You could get flavored water, but wait, 120 calories for raspberry flavored water? You put that back. You could get a regular soft drink for all those calories.

You read the label on a diet soft drink. Zero fat, zero calories, it must be good for me. The beautiful people in the soda commercials say that I can drink all I want of this stuff, right? Think again.

What exactly is in a soft drink? Look at the ingredients. If you drink too much of this stuff, what do you think happens to the chemicals and substances that your body has no use for? They build up and pollute your system over time. You put back the soda and choose something that really quenches your thirst—cold, fresh, pure water, hopefully distilled or spring water from a reputable source.

It seems ironic that we should have to spend as much money on water as we do in today's world, when tap water is so readily available and usually free. The truth is, it is difficult to know just how pure any water is and knowing what type to drink can be very confusing. Our household normally goes through about a five gallon bottle of water on an average of every two or three days.

We normally purchase distilled water, which is supposedly more highly regulated than spring water, which can come from just about any spring anywhere and be labeled as such. Distilled water has gone through a process that breaks it down to only H20 (hydrogen and oxygen) so it inherently lacks nutrients and minerals.

For this reason, we sometimes switch off to spring water, which is reputed to be from a good source, but in reality, one never really knows for certain. I would like to see more stringent regulation on drinking water and have tried various filters and systems but still do not trust the tap water in our area. It seems like a smarter choice to me to choose distilled or spring water over one simply labeled as drinking water from who knows where.

Your level of health is a direct result of the choices that you make on a daily basis. Like a flower or tree nourished by fresh spring rains, your body is a living organism that thrives on plenty of pure water. It is up to you to supply it with what it needs to function at its fullest potential.

Please keep in mind that in praising the benefits of pure water, I am certainly not recommending that you never again have a cup of coffee, soda, glass of wine, or bottle of beer. It would be hypocritical of me to do so. Likewise, in encouraging the pure life path, I am not suggesting that you eat only foods that you have grown yourself on an organic farm, located at the top of an isolated mountain in a nuclear free country. I gave up on that kind of idealistic thinking many years ago.

Perhaps you have encountered people who go to extremes, bordering on unhealthy obsession while striving to be healthy. Along the way, they often lose their zest for life and becoming frustrated while trying to create an impossibly perfect world. Like chronic dieters, they often just give up and fall back into their previous unhealthy patterns, going from one extreme to another.

By using the Pura Vida Stepping stones, you can avoid the pitfall of lifestyle extremes and choose instead to create a healthy, balanced, high quality lifestyle. It is not necessary to feel guilty when you have an occasional lazy day or eat or drink something that is not good for you.

What is important is the state of your overall lifestyle and the daily decisions that you make on a regular, long-term basis. As you know, it is not what you do occasionally that determines the state of your health, but rather, the choices that you make on a consistent basis.

Fortunately, drinking plenty of pure H$_2$O on a consistent basis is one of the easiest things that you can do to improve the function of your body and the state of your health. If only everything else in life were that simple!

Eating For Content

As a nation of impressionable consumers, we all too often accept the advertisements we see on television or in magazines as the truth, subconsciously storing the information as fact because *they* said so without ever questioning the source. Exactly who are the all powerful and all knowing *they* anyway?

When shopping for food to fuel our busy lifestyles, we all need to ask ourselves, "What exactly is in this so-called healthy food product, camouflaged in this subliminally attractive package? Is this product labeled healthy simply because the manufacturers have added some bran, even though it might be full of simple sugars, fat, salt, preservatives, additives, and chemicals?"

Many food manufacturers are more concerned with running a profitable business than they are with supplying their customers with ideal nutritional content in their products. The manufacturers merely give consumers what they demand. It is our way of thinking and purchasing that dictates the practices of the food industry, often resulting in nutritionally empty food products.

If you have already started asking yourself more questions about the everyday products that you purchase, good for you! You are one of the powerful consumers who have recently had a positive influence on the food industry, resulting in changes in labeling and a wider selection of wholesome, nutritious products. Eating well is much easier today than it was a few years ago because of these changes.

As you proceed along your Pura Vida journey, your body requires plenty of high quality fuel to supply you with energy and keep all of its systems running in peak condition. The old adage "You are what you eat" still rings true today. These are just a few of the reasons why the next stepping stone on your Pura Vida Journey involves eating high quality food.

__Stepping stone # 7__: Eat for the nutritional value of your food, not simply for instant gratification.

To truly live up to your Pure Life potential, you need to begin looking at everything that you eat in a whole new way. Your everyday journey through life is full of rituals that are connected with food. Hotdogs at baseball games, birthday cakes, popcorn at the movies, and a big, overstuffed Thanksgiving meal with all the trimmings are just a few of the foods that are often associated with happy memories. It is possible, however, to simply eat reasonable portions of these foods associated with fun or find a healthy substitute for these traditional favorites and still have just as good of a time.

Occasionally eating something that is less than nutritious is a normal part of a healthy lifestyle. Habitual emotional eating, however, can cause a person to veer off of the path of optimal health, and become dependent on certain types of unhealthy food for comfort. Too often, people eat not because they are hungry, but because they are bored, depressed, lonely, or under stress.

When you truly love and respect your body, you will find that you want to nourish it with the proper foods. You will focus your energy on loving your body more than you love certain types of foods.

You will know that you have changed your mindset when you start to realize that many of the choices that you formerly viewed as sacrifices were not really sacrifices at all. Turning down that fatty dessert when you are already full is not denying yourself. You are rewarding yourself, even though it may not feel like it at the time.

You are rewarding yourself by not having to suffer the long-term health consequences of those few moments of instant gustatory gratification. You are really denying yourself when you do not take time to eat well enough to supply your body with the proper fuel it needs to keep running at its peak potential.

As you stand on this seventh solid stepping stone, taking time to gain a fresh, new perspective, it becomes more apparent to you that there is not one single thing that causes one to be unhealthy or overweight. Poor nutritional health often has as much to do with the problems a person may be having in their relationships or at work as it does with the fast food that he or she ate for lunch.

Many overweight people fill their life with food because they are trying to fill a void created by lack of attention, affection, excitement, or meaning in their life. By dealing with the underlying causes, they often discover that being overweight was not the problem. It was merely a symptom representing a general imbalance in their bodies or in their lifestyles.

Take some time right now to honestly examine the way you feel about food. Do you think of food as quality fuel for your body, or do you eat simply for the pleasure and comforting feelings you associate with certain types of food?

Since the quality of your energy level is affected by the type and quality of the food that you eat, cleaning up your diet automatically improves your level of pure, high quality energy. As you know, your daily decisions shape the state of your current and future health. The next time you are making a decision about what to eat, keep the word *nourishment* in mind. After all, that is what food is really for—nourishing your body and keeping it strong, healthy, and loaded with pure energy!

Why Diets Simply Do Not Work

Hopefully, we are all aware enough by now to know that quick fix or severe caloric restriction diets simply do not work, and that they can be very unhealthy and dangerous.

When you severely restrict the amount of calories that you take in, your body perceives this condition as starvation. The body's natural response to starvation is to lighten the load by shedding its muscle tissue. Since muscle is metabolically active, your body needs less food to survive when muscle tissue is lost.

If you are practically starving yourself in order to watch the numbers go down on the scales, remember this; the weight you may lose at first on an extremely low-calorie diet is not only bodyfat. Much of it is muscle, and when muscle tissue is lost, it is actually easier for the body to store fat.

Also, when a person loses muscle tissue, they eventually become weak and tired, resulting in a reduced level of physical activity. In turn, this inactivity and weakness causes an even greater loss of muscle tissue.

Metabolism is the amazing process that converts food (think fuel) to the pure energy that keeps your body going. The innate intelligence of your body efficiently and automatically transforms the food that you eat into the pure energy that you rely on to fuel your busy day through the miracle of metabolism.

Not eating enough food actually slows down the metabolic rate, which is the speed at which your body burns calories. The most metabolically active tissue in your body is muscle. Muscle even burns calories while you are asleep. To put it simply, the more lean muscle you have, the more efficiently your body can burn fat, and the less likely it is that your body will store fat.

Since the process of digestion and absorption takes energy, every time you eat a meal your metabolic rate increases. One of the reasons why eating breakfast is so important is that it kicks in your metabolism early in the day. Also, when you eat smaller, more frequent meals during the day, your metabolic rate naturally rises.

There is no such thing as healthy dieting involving severe caloric restriction. Yes, people do temporarily lose bodyweight on crash diets, but usually end up gaining it back. Keep in mind, however, that there is a major difference between losing bodyweight and losing bodyfat. Vital muscle, water, protein, and glycogen can all account for rapid bodyweight loss. Beware of any program promising that you will lose more than two pounds per week, and always consider the long term negative effects of fad diets on your health.

When I first began studying nutrition, I was surprised to learn that a calorie is not an actual component of food. According to the Merriam-Webster dictionary, the official definition of the term calorie is: the amount of heat required to raise the temperature of one kilogram of water one degree Celsius. Put more simply, the calorie is simply a measure used to express the heat or energy value of food and physical activity. Once again, the mysterious concept of energy, which is intrinsically related to the pure life force flowing through us all, weaves through the course of our daily existence.

Your energy level is affected by every aspect of your lifestyle, but an imbalance in your nutritional energy input usually has the most noticeable and immediate effects on your overall health and well being.

If you are not taking in adequate calories from the right sources, it is impossible to have sufficient energy to lead an active, healthy lifestyle. For this reason, chronic dieters are usually chronically tired. People who are always on a diet rarely have the energy to exercise enough to maintain a healthy ratio of lean muscle to body fat. Eventually, due to uncontrollable hunger, weakness, and frustration, the chronic dieter usually regains the weight lost, and in many cases, gains back even more bodyfat than when they first began dieting.

Chronic rapid weight loss and subsequent gains increase vulnerability to colds and disease, since the body is not supplied with adequate nutrients to strengthen the immune system. What is sometimes referred to as yo-yo dieting has also been linked to menstrual problems and cardiovascular disease.

Over the years, I have seen the harmful physical and emotional effects of chronic dieting in countless individuals and patients. I have also seen many people who are taking potentially dangerous cholesterol medications eat anything they want, mistakenly believing that the medications are a free ticket with no long term consequences. During the peak of the much hyped carb craze, thousands of individuals increased their risk of serious cardiovascular diseases by eating trendy, high fat, low carb diets with little nutritional value. All because the nutritional experts at the time told us it was the right thing to do.

I have personally witnessed hundreds of others frustration with trying to follow complicated diets that are impossible to adhere to in the real world. Often, these experiences adversely affect the dieter's relationships with loved ones and sometimes endanger their lives or cause permanent physical damage.

In the many years that it has taken me to write this guidebook, dozens of books touting the latest, hottest diet have flown on and off of the best seller lists. Historically speaking, that is nothing new. What is newsworthy, however, is that during the past few years there has also been an increase in the number of books and programs that educate the public and teach individuals to think for themselves.

From a broader perspective, in has been encouraging for me to see the recent gradual, positive changes in health consciousness in the overall population. More people are truly beginning to understand that the only way to maintain their own individual, ideal, healthy weight and shape is to make positive, permanent changes in their overall lifestyle. They have had enough of grapefruit diets, magic bullet pills, toning machines, creams, and wraps all promising to melt off the cellulite. They have finally come to understand that the bottom line is maintaining a healthy balance in their life.

They are also realizing that, for every person featured in ridiculous before and after weight loss scams, there are hundreds of thousands who have lost bodyfat the common sense way. They are accepting the fact that if it sounds too good to be true, it probably is. They are also recognizing the fact that millions of people maintain healthy physiques and lifestyles naturally, without the expensive help of trendy opportunists.

By learning the facts and using common sense, you can permanently lose excess bodyfat without starving yourself. If you are sick and tired of all the hype and nonsense surrounding weight loss, perhaps it is time to return to the basics.

Be completely honest with yourself as you step back and look at the entire picture of your current lifestyle. Spend time engaging in activities that will nourish and connect your mind, body, and spirit and create a more balanced, healthy way of living on a day-to-day basis.

Rather than using discipline as a short term, negative tool in order to starve yourself, use it in a positive, long-term way to create a healthier, more energetic lifestyle. Let your positive intentions and desires work in your favor as you allow your inner voice to guide you along a healthier, more fulfilling path.

If, in the past, you have felt like a prisoner trapped in your own body, and suffered countless disappointments with countless diets, make a conscious decision to liberate yourself by changing your course, seeking your own truth, and truly becoming the master of your own destiny.

Pure Fuel

I have always been fascinated by the intricate metabolic process that enables our intelligent bodies to take the food that we supply them with and transform that fuel into the energy that we need to get through our busy days. In essence, the quality and amount of energy that we have depends largely on the quality and amount of the food that we eat.

It is a simple fact of life that your body's most basic need is for energy. To obtain this energy it requires two things: food as its fuel and oxygen to burn this fuel. To supply your body with the pure energy it needs to function at its fullest potential, you must provide it with the proper amount and the proper type of fuel or nutrients.

There are six different types of nutrients: proteins, carbohydrates, fats, vitamins, minerals, and water. Only proteins, carbohydrates, and fats, which are considered macronutrients, are a direct source of energy, however. The other three nutrients are indirectly involved in providing your body with energy.

When it comes to the process of metabolism, all calories are not the same. It is important to remember that your body does not process all of the calories derived from these macronutrient sources in the same way. Dietary fat turns into body fat easily because fat calories can be stored immediately in the fat cells basically as they are. For example, if you ate a fast food cheeseburger and fries for lunch, the calories coming from fat in this meal require very little processing before settling on your hips, thighs, stomach or other fat storage depot.

The remaining calories in that meal coming from carbohydrates and protein require much more energy to be processed and thus are less likely to be stored as fat and more likely to be used as energy.

If you decided, however, to have protein and complex carbohydrate rich beans and brown rice, grilled chicken or a mixed green salad for lunch, this meal is less likely to turn into bodyfat, because it takes considerably more energy to digest and break down the complex carbohydrates and protein from a meal such as this, than it does from a meal that is high in saturated fat.

Fortunately, you do not have to shuffle through life shaking with weakness, while your stomach protests noisily, in order to lose weight. You can actually eat more and still lose excess bodyfat if you are eating the proper kinds of foods. It is neither healthy nor smart to place yourself on a strict, low-calorie diet, in which you end up weak, frustrated, undernourished, and consistently hungry.

Making well-informed nutritional choices is easier today than it has ever been, if you educate yourself, use common sense, and stay away from fad diets and trendy weight loss products. Instead of spending your valuable time and hard earned money on useless gimmicks, why not really invest it in your health? Invest that money in organic fruits and vegetables for yourself and your family. Invest that precious time in exercising your body, and improving the quality of your health and overall well-being.

As you begin to adopt the Pura Vida lifestyle, you will find that you naturally develop a preference for fresh, living foods. You may also find that you eventually lose the cravings for foods that are pumped full of salt, sugar, fats, and chemicals.

When you lead a more balanced, fulfilling lifestyle, you will discover that your emotion-based cravings for certain foods diminish. When you allow your innate intelligence to have a part in the decision making process, you will find yourself naturally avoiding foods with empty calories and instead, choosing ones with high nutritional content, fiber, and energy potential.

Anyone who has ever proudly harvested fruits and vegetables that they have grown themselves can appreciate the time, energy, and proper conditions that growing live foods requires. As a result of watching and nurturing their gardens, gardeners instinctively know that there is a life force that makes fresh, living foods superior to those that are produced in a factory.

For me, gardening is a hobby that does more than reduce stress and provide me with a distraction from the concerns of everyday life. Activities such as digging in the dirt and pruning the leaves of the hundreds of banana trees that I have planted in my yard over the years keeps me moving and helps me stay in shape. Enjoying the tasty fruits of my labor and sharing them with others is a thrill that makes all those hours of sweating in the hot sun and shoveling holes worthwhile. Gardening and working in the yard also helps me connect with the earth and keeps me a little more grounded than simply going for a walk or swimming in the ocean does.

At the peak of my gardening days, when I was much younger and more energetic, I once canned thirty-six quarts of salsa, using only fresh tomatoes, onions, various types of peppers, and garlic that I had grown myself in a much loved and nurtured organic garden in West Virginia. I truly believe that the fruits of my labor helped improve the health of everyone who enjoyed them that fall. Who knows? Perhaps the antioxidants even helped fight off a virus or two.

For me, there is something very exciting and somewhat spiritual about picking an apple from a tree branch and biting into a juicy, delicious food that was connected to a living tree, with its roots firmly planted in the rich brown soil of the earth only seconds before. This apple truly is a perfect food in that it contains the seeds of future pure life and energy within itself.

Many of our Costa Rican friends seemed to innately understand the importance of eating fresh, whole foods and, in some ways, were more nutritionally advanced than some of our country's so called experts. They knew that time spent tending their family gardens, connecting with the earth, and preparing and eating sit-down meals with their close-knit families was time very well spent.

Their attitudes, expressions, and lifestyles reflected this pure life energy resulting from their choices and lifestyle decisions. In this era of bio-engineered food and eating on the run, we could all benefit by following their example and including more wholesome, real food in our daily diets.

There are times when I wonder if a family that we met in Costa Rica (who we fondly remember as the Volcano Family) had the right idea. We met this delightfully innocent family after a coincidental encounter with their friend Donald, who rented us two very high-spirited, mountain-bred horses for the day.

After an exhilarating and very long horseback ride through the jungle, Donald led us to the family's simple wooden home, which was perched on top of a verdant, misty mountain, complete with a stunning view of the Arenal Volcano. We witnessed extraordinary glimpses of a much simpler way of life along the steep path, including children using giant leaves as umbrellas during a warm and gentle rain shower.

The Volcano Family invited us into their home and lives with open arms, sharing their simple, home grown food with such a generosity of spirit, wide eyed curiosity, and a feeling of unconditional love that we were truly amazed and pleasantly surprised.

The three small, yet exuberant Volcano Family boys were barefoot and playing soccer in the field near their board and batten house when we arrived. It seemed to us that they literally radiated good health and positive energy as we approached them on horseback and tied our horses next to the mule that seemed to be the family's only means of transportation.

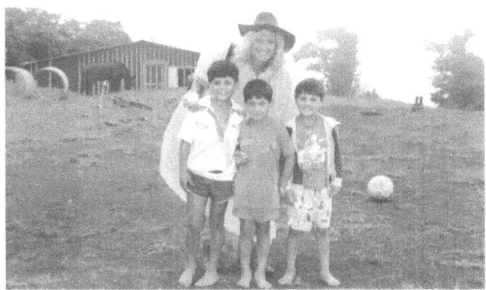

This sincere and genuine family lived farther away from civilization than any-one we have ever met and their home was accessible only on horseback or by walking miles on foot. Yet, in some ways they were more evolved than us.

The Volcano Family grew most of their own food in the nutrient rich soil of their garden, got plenty of exercise in the surrounding wilderness, and were openly trusting and affectionate. Their tiny house literally overflowed with laugh-ter and joy.

Watching them stand in the rustic doorway, waving goodbye, with the *Vulcan Arenal* as the backdrop, we were left with a lasting impression of the true Pura Vida spirit. This moving experience caused something inside of us to shift a little, and somehow pointed us in a different direction. As the bright eyed boys impul-sively escorted us partway down the mountain and presented us with a hand woven gift, we could not help but feel blessed and realize that we are all on this journey together.

At that moment, I can remember clearly thinking that the life force responsi-ble for creating the corn or beans that any of us eats for dinner is the same pure energy that circulates around the Volcano Family's garden and loving home. We all gaze at the same stars at night and are bathed in the light of the same sun and moon.

On another level, by making family, friends, and faith a higher priority than possessions and consumerism, simple people such as these seem to have discov-ered a truth that it takes some of us a lifetime to realize.

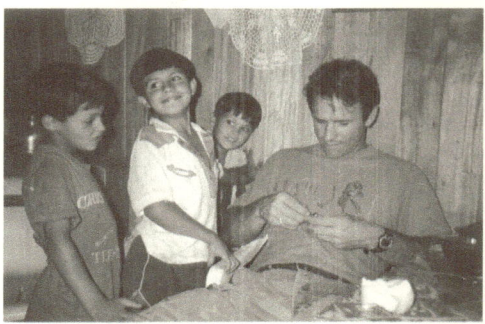

There is a reason why fresh, whole food is so good for us that cannot be explained with scientific jargon and clinical, corporate sponsored research studies. It has to do with a mysterious, intangible, elusive force that causes volcanoes to erupt and children to run, play, and grow. In essence, it is the miracle of life itself. Real food, real life, real energy, Pura Vida!

Fiber And Whole Foods

"Eat mostly fresh vegetables, fruits, whole grains, and legumes, and drink more water." You have been hearing this for years, but have you ever truly tried it on a long-term basis? Have you ever really experienced what it feels like to eat mostly whole, natural foods? It is remarkable how including more fresh, whole foods in your diet makes such a noticeable difference in your overall health and pure energy level.

It is fairly safe to say that only a small percentage of the United States' population has heeded this advice. I wish I could say that I was a full time member of this group, but I have my rebellious, backsliding days, just like most people. Somewhere deep in the recesses of my subconscious, however, is a little voice (I sometimes think of it as an inborn GPS) that always tries to steer me back in the right direction.

One thing that I have found particularly helpful is starting my grocery shopping in the produce department. After selecting all of the fresh fruits and vegetables that I think we will realistically eat, the frugal part of me is less likely to add extra snacks and junk to my shopping cart. By reversing the normal order of grocery shopping, I also try to find foods that will compliment the veggie choices that I have made rather than thinking of them as a side dish.

I am fortunate because I live near several excellent health food stores and year round fresh fruit and vegetable markets. As often as possible, I enjoy loading up on fresh tomatoes, corn, green peppers, green beans, strawberries, apples, oranges, and other assorted goodies. Perhaps you live in an area that has a farmer's market on the weekends or an awesome produce market that will provide a similar experience. At one of my favorite local markets, the owners often provide me with a huge box that I fill up with goodies, including fresh herb plants and homemade breads.

When the weather and our traveling schedule permits, I supplement this produce with vegetables and herbs from our own small organic garden. There is actually a growing school of thought that is based on the concept that eating foods grown close to where you live is better for you. I find that philosophy very interesting and have just started to research the idea.

There is no feeling in the world quite like watching a plant sprout from a tiny seed and grow into a nourishing fruit or vegetable. You can almost feel the pure life energy circulating through a freshly picked tomato. Perhaps that is part of the reason that no matter how much processed foods are synthetically fortified with vitamins and minerals, they never have quite the same positive physiological effects on your body as fresh, whole foods.

If you cannot remember the last time you ate a juicy peach, strawberry, or piece of watermelon, maybe it is time to give them another try. Life's simple pleasures truly are the best. Perhaps more importantly, by eating a variety of vegetables and fruits on a daily basis you may also be decreasing your risk of many types of cancer, including lung, prostate, and stomach cancers.

About ten years ago, our local supermarket added a very small organic fruit and vegetable section, another example of industry responding to the consumers' demands. The organic section has expanded significantly since that time. I interpret this and similar changes as a positive sign that our society's collective health consciousness is being raised, and that the current interest in health and nutrition is not simply another passing trend.

With the growing popularity of large franchise natural health food stores such as Wild Oats and Whole Foods Market, organic foods are gradually making their way into mainstream America. The fact that celebrities are often photographed shopping at these type of stores seems to have increased the coolness factor and made organic food more appealing to some.

Organically grown foods are more expensive and sometimes harder to find, but they are usually worth the extra cost and effort. Try fitting them into your budget by cutting back on meats full of saturated fat or unhealthy snacks and beverages. You may not be able to see or even taste it, but there is a significant difference.

Most processed, packaged foods lack fiber, a key element that is absolutely necessary for the digestive system to function efficiently. The more refined and processed a food is, the less fiber it usually contains.

Fiber is plant material that cannot be digested by your body. It adds bulk to waste material and helps move it through the digestive tract, sweeping the colon clean in the process. Fiber is found naturally in abundance in fruits and vegetables such as corn, peas, potatoes, broccoli, carrots, citrus fruits, apples, bananas, and figs. Other excellent sources are whole grains, such as brown rice and steel cut or old fashioned oats, and legumes.

The list of lean fibrous vegetables, which provide plenty of fiber and minerals, is almost endless. Celery and green leafy vegetables (the darker green, the better) are especially good at sweeping wastes out of the system. Spinach, kale, collard greens, and cabbage are all good sources of fiber.

Inadequate fiber intake is thought to be a contributing factor in colon cancer, a leading cause of death in America. The typical American consumes only about half of the twenty-five grams of fiber recommended for every two thousand calories eaten. Excessive fiber intake is not recommended however, because a level that is extremely high could decrease the absorption of calcium, iron, magnesium, phosphorous, and certain trace minerals.

It is amazing that many people consider not going to the bathroom for two or three days to be normal. Your digestive system was designed to eliminate waste material on a daily basis. When sluggish digestion and constipation occur, toxins and wastes are not being flushed out by the normal process of elimination. Your whole body can become toxic if your digestive system is not regular, often resulting in loss of energy, headaches, and bloating.

Many people reach for habit-forming laxatives to quickly fix the condition of constipation rather than making an effort to do something about the cause of the problem. Long-term abuse of laxatives can be dangerous because the nerves that cause the colon to contract and move waste products through the digestive system can be damaged over time. The colon eventually relies on laxatives to do the work and can lose its normal contractile action.

One or two prunes a day or some bran on your cereal is helpful, but usually not enough to help keep your system running smoothly. In order to aid your digestive system's natural process of elimination, it is necessary to increase your consumption of lean fibrous vegetables and whole grains, drink more water, and get plenty of exercise.

Drinking plenty of water is essential in helping to move waste material though the colon because water helps give fiber its bulk. Exercise also helps speed up the transit time of the digestive system. If you have tried all of the suggestions listed above and still have problems with elimination, an herb called cascara sagrada may give you temporary relief and is safer than over the counter medications such as Ex-lax.

Most refined products have been stripped of bran, the fiber rich husk found in whole grains. When you eat foods such as cereal, rice, and breads that are made from whole grains, you naturally increase the amount of bran in your diet. Although bran has little or no nutritional value, it is important nonetheless because it absorbs water as it moves through the colon and can help speed up bowel movements.

One slice of whole wheat bread, which is rich in bran, contains three and one-half times more fiber than a slice of white bread. One-half of a cup of brown rice contains five times more fiber than an equal amount of white rice, which has been stripped of its bran husk.

Recently, the FDA released some good news for a change. It confirmed the first food-specific health claim to be used on labels: that soluble fiber from oatmeal, as part of a low saturated fat, low cholesterol diet, may reduce the risk of heart disease.

Steel cut or old fashioned, organic oats have been a staple in our personal daily diet for many years. For some time now, we have been eating organic uncooked oats lightly sprinkled with Grape Nuts and sometimes honey, raisins, or bananas in skim or rice milk for breakfast. Although we normally try to eat a variety of different types of foods for breakfast, this unique item is often on our early morning menu.

I often add a small amount of some sort of nuts, such as walnuts on days when I know that I am going to be particularly busy and need extra energy. This concoction may not appeal to everyone's taste buds and has certainly raised the eyebrows of many of our friends and members of our family.

The funny thing is, however, that many of the people who we dared to eat this unique mixture have included it in their morning routine after finding that it tastes better than it looks. Like us, they have also found that this quick breakfast in a bowl provides them with plenty of fiber and an exceptionally high level of lasting energy for their busy mornings.

The soluble fiber found in unrefined oat products, citrus fruits, apples, and beans is thought to help prevent heart disease by lowering blood cholesterol. Soluble fiber acts like a sponge, soaking up water as it moves through the colon, resulting in larger, softer stools.

Currently, there is some disagreement as to whether or not the other type of fiber, known as insoluble fiber found in wheat bran, brown rice, nuts, and thoroughly washed, unpeeled vegetables lowers the risk of colorectal cancer. Personally, I believe it does. This controversy should not stop you from making an effort to obtain enough fiber in your diet, however, since fiber does have other important functions in the digestive system.

Proper digestion and elimination are affected by many factors, including nutrition, your water intake, your activity level, and even your emotional state—yet another excellent example of how everything in your body is interrelated and interdependent. By applying the experience and knowledge that you have gained from utilizing the previous stepping stones, you can increase your odds of maintaining a healthy digestive system, directly affecting the function of every other system of your body.

By listening to your body, choosing foods with high nutritional content, drinking plenty of pure water, and preventing and reducing the negative effects of stress in your life, you will create a cleaner, healthier internal environment, which positively affects your outer appearance and the quality of your life. If you don't believe that factors such as stress affect your appearance, take a look at photos of your loved ones when they are exceptionally happy and smiling. To me, a heartfelt laugh or smile is the most attractive anti-aging medicine that we possess.

The collective power of the stepping stones creates an awesome force that I like to call *Pure Momentum*. This is one of the most powerful principles of the Pura Vida philosophy, instinctively practiced by the ancient builders of the Pure Life path. The next stepping stone is strategically placed near the top of a steep hill, which can only be reached as a result of consistent forward momentum.

Stepping Stone # 8: *Maintaining a strong, steady level of pure momentum is the eighth stepping stone along your personal path of optimal health and well being.*

You have likely experienced the positive effects of healthy momentum along your own voyage through life and already know what a noticeable difference it makes in the quality of your life. Pure Momentum is created by a combination of healthy choices and actions which all contribute to steady forward movement along the right path. Regardless of the obstacles facing you along the way, you can plow straight through them once you have established a consistently strong and steady momentum.

When you repeatedly make wrong choices, however, you eventually lose your Pure Momentum and may end up progressing slowly, with frequent, erratic stops and starts. Like every other aspect of your Pura Vida lifestyle, Pure Momentum is composed of a healthy balance of each integral component of the Pure Life Triune.

A clear, focused mind, a strong, well fueled body, and an energized, connected spirit are essential to getting and keeping the ball rolling. This is the key not only to living your life to its fullest potential at this very moment, but also to forming the foundation for the dynamic momentum that keeps you joyfully and steadily moving forward.

This pure momentum provides you with the high quality energy that easily carries you over the next hill or obstacle into the future and to the next exciting chapter of your unique Pura Vida Journey. The adventure is just beginning.

Complex Carbohydrates: Pure Energy Fuel

Has this ever happened to you? You were in a hurry and skipped breakfast six hours ago, and now you are at work, running errands, or stuck in traffic. You feel that if you do not eat something—anything—very soon, you cannot be held responsible for your own actions.

We have all felt ourselves becoming increasingly irritable, shaky, and weak when we go too long without eating. This is simply because we do not have any fuel left to supply our bodies with energy. Our gas tanks are on empty.

If someone told you that there was a natural pill that you could take that would provide you with plenty of consistent energy throughout your busy day, you probably would be eager to buy it. Fortunately, that miracle product is available at your local grocery or health food store—except it does not come in pill form. This magic substance, that I like to call pure energy fuel, is actually a macronutrient, specifically complex carbohydrates, and is found in a wide variety of wholesome, natural foods.

When you hear people talking about carbs, it is very important to keep in mind that not all carbohydrates are created the same. There are two basic types of carbohydrates: simple sugars (such as those found in fruits and table sugar) and complex carbohydrates, which are found in whole grain foods and vegetables.

Complex carbohydrates provide you with a more sustained level of consistent energy and do not turn into bodyfat as easily as simple sugars or dietary fat. Both simple sugars and complex carbohydrates are changed into glucose (blood sugar) during digestion to provide an immediate source of energy. The glucose that is not used right away is stored as glycogen in the liver and muscles. When your body does not have enough of these glycogen stores, your muscles are weak and you lack energy.

When you begin to exercise, your primary energy source is carbohydrates. During exercise, the carbohydrates stored as muscle glycogen are used as a source of energy for the specific muscle in which they are stored. A diet high in complex carbohydrates actually increases the capacity of the muscles to store glycogen.

One of the major differences between the two types of carbohydrates is that simple sugars, in contrast to complex carbohydrates, are released quickly into the system. This release gives you a quick burst of energy often called a sugar rush, which is usually followed by an unpleasant crash.

Refined sugars, such as ordinary white table sugar, are considered empty calorie foods because they supply only energy in the form of calories with little or no nutritional value. Simple carbohydrates, such as those found in sugary snacks, are more easily converted into bodyfat than complex carbohydrates, such as those carbs found in whole grains. Eating too many simple sugars can also adversely affect your body's hunger mechanism, blocking the hormones such as leptin which tells you "Okay, I am full, you can stop eating now."

Simple carbohydrates are constructed of either single (mono) or double (di) molecules of sugar called monosaccharides and disaccharides. On the other hand, most complex carbohydrates are nutrient rich and the energy that they provide is released more evenly, providing you with more consistent levels of energy throughout your busy day. Complex carbohydrates, or polysaccharides (poly means many) contain many sugar molecules joined in long chains.

Earlier, I mentioned how important it is to combine your meals properly. When you eat a meal high in complex carbohydrates combined with a moderate amount of lean protein, it will take the digestive system longer to process and break down your meal than it would with a meal that is extremely high in fat.

The good news is that your body will actually burn a considerable amount of calories while processing a meal such as this, whereas most of the calories from a high fat meal are stored immediately as body fat.

Also, it is interesting to note that a certain level of carbohydrate breakdown is necessary for fats to be metabolized for energy. In other words, fats burn in a carbohydrate flame. If your diet is extremely high in proteins and fat but very low in carbohydrates, your body may have difficulty metabolizing fat for energy. This is just one of the many reasons why it is important to include plenty of whole grains, vegetables, and legumes in your daily diet.

Contrary to recent headlines about the complicated pasta controversy, eating pasta and other complex carbohydrates will not automatically make you fat, unless you take in more than your body can use. As with everything else in life, you can get too much of a good thing. One of the downsides to pasta is that traditional white noodles are usually made from ingredients that are lacking in nutrients and fiber.

If you take in more carbohydrates than your body uses, the unused balance is eventually stored as bodyfat. Of course, if you eat a heaping plate of pasta or load it down with creamy sauces and meaty toppings, it will turn into bodyfat if your body does not need the calories for energy.

Pay particular attention to serving sizes on package labels to obtain a more accurate picture of your actual carbohydrate intake. What you think of as a normal serving of cereal, rice, or pasta may actually be considered as two or three servings. Being aware of your true carb intake throughout the day and even writing down or measuring the actual amounts that you consume may help you to avoid overindulging.

Part of the reason that many people have a tendency to keep eating carb rich foods once they start may have to do with the soothing effect these foods can have on your body's chemistry and the way that these foods affect the neurological system once metabolized. This calming effect has to do with neurotransmitters such as serotonin and can be heightened in individuals with biochemical imbalances.

Overindulging in sugars and complex carbs often has to do with emotional links to comforting foods as well as a psychological need to feel full after eating. For many people, processed sugar truly can be a dangerous substance and a direct contributor to diseases such as adult onset diabetes.

Regardless of how one views the ongoing carb addict controversy, the fact remains that there are more than twice as many calories in fat as there are in complex carbohydrates and that many complex carbohydrates, such as those found in vegetables, are an excellent source of nutrition and energy when consumed in balanced moderation.

You can find a wide variety of organic whole wheat, spinach, and vegetable pastas that are more nutrient rich than refined white pasta in some grocery stores and most health food stores. You can also replace traditional refined bagels with lower fat, oat and bran bagels without sacrificing taste.

By choosing brown rice instead of white rice, and whole grain breads over white bread, you are also obtaining more nutrients and fiber in your high-energy food choices. I often buy some of our whole grains and legumes in bulk at the health food store, which is less expensive than buying packaged products.

When doing your grocery shopping this week, remember: energy producing complex carbohydrates are found in whole grains, beans, and vegetables. Some good sources of complex carbohydrates are pinto beans, white beans, kidney beans, garbanzo beans, brown rice, corn, steel cut or old-fashioned oatmeal, peas, potatoes, sweet potatoes, and whole grain rice cakes.

Whole grains, which are actually the seeds of plants, are high in energy producing complex carbohydrates (70–85 percent in most grains). They are also low in fat, and naturally high in protein, fiber, vitamins, and minerals.

The simple sugar sucrose (table sugar) is the main ingredient found in cakes, candy, and other sweets. Try to limit the amount of sucrose in your diet since excessive dietary sugar intake has been linked to diabetes, obesity, coronary heart disease, and tooth decay. Simple sugars are also found in milk (galactose), malt sugar (maltose), and in fruits and fruit juices (fructose).

Because of their high nutrient and fiber content, it is my opinion that fruits and fruit juices should be a regular part of the average person's daily diet. I do feel that fruits and fruit juices should be consumed in moderation, however. Try including more of the not-so-sweet apples (such as Granny Smith) and berry fruits, such as strawberries, blackberries, and blueberries, and fewer grapes and raisins. Bananas are somewhat sweet but they are high in potassium and other vital nutrients.

Many trendy diets forbid eating fruits and vegetables and instead recommend food such as saturated fat filled steaks, eggs, and cheese, and also foods such as MacDonald's Egg McMuffins—all in the name of quick weight loss and muscle building.

Although including plenty of high quality protein in your daily diet is crucial, it is equally as important to eat plenty of fresh, whole, pure life foods that increase your pure energy level and decrease your risk of cardiovascular disease and other health problems. Personally, I believe that some of the facts associated with low carb diets are true, especially those related to the risks of over consumption of sugar and the subsequent disease processes related to excess sugar intake. It is sometimes hard to separate fact from profit producing fiction, however.

In my experience, the meteoric rise and fall of low carb diets was most accurately reflected in the supermarket. The sudden appearance of overpriced and attractively packaged products (mostly containing chemical sugar substitutes) corresponded directly with marketing blitzes and advertising dollars.

When the average consumer attempted to stay on the restrictive diets long term, however, most struggled. Around the time that most dieters were entering a maintenance phase, I remember seeing aisle after aisle of clearance items in the low carb products. I'm sure that the fact that many of the products tasted terrible didn't help much either. The thing that concerned me most about the low carb craze was the associated increased risk of heart disease associated with increased consumption of saturated fats.

If you obtain a large percentage of your daily calories from complex carbohydrates and a moderate amount of protein, rather than fat sources, you will supply your body with cleaner fuel to burn. Complex carbohydrates leave behind fewer by-products after their digestion and require less metabolic work for the internal organs.

Although a moderate amount of protein is essential in your diet, beware of popular diets that are extremely high in protein. The metabolism of excessive dietary protein can damage the liver and kidneys. I will discuss protein in more detail in the next chapter.

Currently, there is some controversy over what percentage of your total calories should be obtained from each macronutrient source. This is a classic example of how society's guidelines and what we accept as fact are constantly fluctuating.

Exactly what percentage of your total calories should come from each of the three sources varies, depending on what you read and to whom you listen. One thing that most nutrition experts do tend to agree on, however, is that carbohydrates should make up the largest portion of your daily calorie consumption.

When you supply your body with a sufficient amount of unrefined complex carbohydrates, you are ensuring that your innately intelligent body will use carbohydrates for fuel and reserve the protein that you consume for building and maintaining muscle. Since muscle requires more calories to sustain itself than fat tissue, the more muscle you have, the more calories you burn during your everyday activities.

The U.S. Food and Drug Administration (FDA) has recently set new daily values (DVs) for important nutrients. Under these new guidelines, it is recommended that about 60% of your total daily caloric intake should come from carbohydrates, 30% or less from fat, and 10% from protein.

Although these guidelines are somewhat helpful, I personally have found that a lower percentage of fat and slightly higher percentage of protein than recommended by the FDA works best to fuel a healthy, active lifestyle.

Since every individual is unique, no two people have exactly the same requirements. Your ideal daily caloric intake depends on many factors, including your current activity level and overall health. All the calculations and charts are only helpful guidelines established for the general population. The new food labels do, however, make it easier to find out how much of your daily value of carbohydrates, fat, and protein is found in one serving of a particular food.

Quite honestly, all of these numbers can be somewhat confusing. The bottom line is that in the real world, the majority of people do not take the time to calculate their actual nutrient consumption percentages on a regular basis. In my opinion, what really matters is that you get the big picture, listen to your body's innate wisdom, and be consistently aware of what you eat as you travel along your own unique, ever changing path.

Rather than throwing your hands in the air after hearing ten different recommendations from ten different experts and constantly juggling conflicting numbers in your mind, take a deep breath, relax, and place your feet solidly on the next important stepping stone. Tread lightly, however, because growing near this irregular shaped stepping stone is a rare purple orchid, which can be only be found in certain remote, unspoiled corners of the world. The rich, dark soil of the earth in these isolated spots has taken centuries to form and has never been stripped of its irreplaceable nutrients and minerals.

The ancient virgin trees and foliage surrounding this exotic orchid allow precisely the right amount of sunlight and water to penetrate and nurture this symbolic plant. The survival and health of this exotic orchid depends on the source and quality of the nutrients that nourish it. When making nutritional decisions along your daily path, ignore all the hype and nonsense and consider the following Stepping Stone.

<u>Stepping Stone # 9</u>: *Keep in mind that the source and quality of your nutrients is equally as important as the amounts.*

It makes a substantial difference whether you obtain your daily allowance of fat from grilled fish that is high in essential nutrients, or from a greasy cheeseburger dripping with saturated fat. This important fact seems to be overlooked all too often in official recommendations and short lived diet programs.

In my experience, I have found that it is most important to be aware of everything that goes into your body, and to pay special attention to the feedback that your body's innate intelligence gives you. The healthier you become, the more sensitive you will be to the signs and symptoms that your body provides you.

The cleaner your diet becomes, the easier it is to find out exactly which foods agree or disagree with your digestive system and which combinations provide you with the most energy. The more in tune you are with your body, the easier it is to hear what it is trying to tell you.

As you naturally evolve and become more aware, your personal health belief system will also evolve and change. As we progress through the new millennium, I believe that the unprecedented amount of information available to us will drastically change the way that we all think about health and nutrition.

As seekers of truth, we all gather, sort through, and add this information to our current belief system, all the while knowing that what we consider to be the truth today will soon change and be reshaped, based on the new information and experiences we acquire in the future.

Information, however, is simply a collection of words and numbers unless you take the time and energy to integrate what you have learned into your daily life-style, and act in accordance with your new belief system. Think for yourself, experiment with, and apply what you have learned, and see how it works specifically for you.

Pure Protein

Lately, one of the three macronutrients has been receiving quite a bit of press, and also more than its fair share of controversy. If you are confused by all of the information and misinformation swirling around concerning dietary protein, perhaps it is a good idea to learn the basic facts about this popular subject and then form your own opinion. As you have found thus far on your Pura Vida journey, the more you know, the easier it is to sort out the truth from the hype.

Since protein is found in every cell of your body, it is a vital nutrient for all bodily functions. In essence, your whole body is made of protein. Dietary protein is found in foods such as meat, chicken, fish, egg whites, beans, and whole grains. Once protein is eaten, it is broken down into amino acids, which are nicknamed the building blocks of protein.

Amino acids provide the main substance for making the components of the cell, as well as new tissue. Disease-fighting antibodies are also formed from these powerful little amino acids. Proteins are also essential for the process of muscle contraction. When you are moving your body, two structural proteins, known as actin and myosin, slide past each other as the muscle shortens.

Amino acids are also necessary for the formation of muscle tissue. I have always found it fascinating that, to build bigger muscles, your body must first break down muscle tissue (during a process called catabolism) and then repair and rebuild muscle (anabolism). Protein is an irreplaceable component of this natural cycle, and is essential for both growth and repair. Serious athletes may require more protein than the average person for this reason.

Now, it gets a little more complicated. There are two types of amino acids found in protein: essential and nonessential. Nonessential amino acids can be produced by the body. Essential amino acids, on the other hand, must be obtained through your diet. Here is how I remember the two types of amino acids: it is essential that you eat foods containing essential amino acids. Proteins that contain the essential amino acids can be found in foods of both plant and animal origins.

Proteins containing reasonable amounts of all the essential amino acids in the correct ratios to allow for tissue growth and repair are known as complete proteins. Some of the proteins coming from animal sources, such as poultry, meat, fish, milk, and eggs are considered complete proteins for this reason.

Proteins lacking ideal amounts of one or more of the essential amino acids are considered incomplete proteins. Vegetable proteins such as dried beans, lentils, peas, nuts, and cereals are classified as incomplete for this reason.

The fact that certain vegetable proteins are considered incomplete does not necessarily mean that there is something better about a specific amino acid from an animal source as compared to the same amino acid from a vegetable source. It simply means that incomplete protein from a single plant source, when eaten by itself, does not contain every one of the essential amino acids.

By eating a wide variety of foods such as grains, legumes, and vegetables, each providing a different quantity and quality of amino acids, it is possible to obtain all of the essential amino acids. The proteins from plant sources provide more nutritional benefits when eaten in certain combinations. Throughout history, there have always been traditional favorites in most cultures that naturally contain complementary amino acids. For example, beans and rice, a staple in many cultures throughout the world, contain complementary amino acids.

Some good sources of protein from plant sources are nuts and seeds, whole grains such as rice, oats, barley, and whole wheat, and legumes, such as lentils, soybeans, peas, and dried beans. The key word here is variety.

Infants, children, the elderly, and breast-feeding or pregnant women require more protein than others. Stress, injury, and disease may also increase the body's protein requirements. Insufficient dietary protein can cause a lack of energy, stunted growth, and increased chance of disease, due to a weakened immune system. Starvation diets can result in a protein deficiency and accompanying loss of muscle tissue.

When you eat a meal that is high in protein, your metabolic rate rises significantly. Since protein is an essential element of metabolism, an inadequate dietary protein intake makes it harder for your body to burn fat.

The proper combination of a relatively high level of complex carbohydrates and moderate amount of protein in your diet produces a slow, steady release of energy. However, as with all foods, if you eat more protein than your body needs, it will eventually be converted to bodyfat.

Protein is necessary to form lean muscle. It is important to remember, however, that your amount of lean muscle does not increase if you consume more protein than your body requires for energy. The size of the muscle depends on the physical demands made upon it, rather than the extra amount of protein in the diet. In other words, simply eating a lot of protein is not automatically going to make you more muscular.

Consuming excessive amounts of dietary protein can actually be harmful because the metabolism of large quantities of protein can place a strain on liver and kidney function, contributing to dehydration, electrolyte imbalance, and actual muscle tissue loss.

In addition, trendy high protein diets often consist of large amounts of red meat, which is high in artery clogging saturated fat and cholesterol. It is not necessary to rely heavily on red meat for your daily protein requirements. Due largely to over consumption of red meat, the average American consumes twice the amount of protein recommended. Again, the source of your nutrients is equally as important as the percentage.

The skinless white meat of chicken and turkey is a high quality protein that is also a good source of vitamins and minerals. These meats are an excellent source of protein, relatively low in fat, and full of vitamins and minerals. Protein rich fish is the best source of omega-3 fatty acids, which can help prevent the plaque buildup that contributes to cardiovascular disease.

Protein is simply one of the six essential nutrients that are vital for optimal health. The other five nutrients (carbohydrates, fats, vitamins, minerals, and water) are equally as important. Protein is not the single magic bullet that some marketing specialists would like us to believe.

Protein is, however, a vital nutrient necessary for all bodily functions, including the formation of muscle tissue, and creating the components of the cell and disease fighting antibodies. What is truly amazing is how the building blocks of protein join together in an intricate process that makes life as we know it possible.

The real magic is performed when your incredibly intelligent body takes the high quality, clean protein that you supply it with and creates new living tissue. This is the truly miraculous power of protein, but then again, every nutrient and every organ and system of your body is miraculous, and each is equally important. This is the simple beauty of pure life itself.

The Truth About Dietary Fats

An Aussie friend of mine once told me that she never had any problem with her weight until she moved to the United States. She had been raised in the Australian countryside, eating mostly fresh vegetables and whole grains, and was shocked to see how much of the typical American diet consists of fatty fast foods and fried or buttery dishes.

In this land of plenty, the average American diet still far exceeds the recommended percentage of total calories from fat, despite the recent flood of information about the importance of reducing dietary fat.

The American Heart Association and the National Cholesterol Education program both recommend that your diet should be limited to no more than 30% of calories from fats, and, of that, saturated fats should not exceed 10%. The key words here are no more than and not exceeding.

Since cardiovascular disease is now the number one killer not only of men but of women in this country, it is imperative for us all to know the facts about dietary factors affecting heart disease. Because women have a tendency to experiment with popular diets more than men, they should particularly be aware of health risks associated with following trendy high fat diets on a long term basis.

One should never ignore the fact that some dietary fat is required for optimal health. Without adequate amounts of fat in your diet, your body would not be able to make certain vitamins available for use. Dietary fat serves as a carrier for the fat soluble vitamins A, D, E and K. Consequently, a significant reduction of fat from the diet can lead to vitamin deficiency.

In addition, there are some fats, known as essential fatty acids or EFAs that are necessary for proper functioning of the body. These EFAs have a protective effect on the body and can only be obtained through the diet. Some good sources of EFAs are safflower oil, canola oil, flaxseed oil, and evening primrose oil.

Just as amino acids are the building blocks of protein, fatty acids are the building blocks of fats. Fatty acids are classified as either saturated or unsaturated. There are two types of unsaturated fats; monounsaturated and polyunsaturated.

Just in case you are starting to become a little confused by all of these monos, dis, and polys, here is a quick review. Mono means one, di means two, and poly means many. Saccharide refers to sugars or carbohydrates. Monosaccharides and disaccharides are the two types of simple sugars or carbohydrates. Complex carbohydrates, or polysaccharides, contain many sugar molecules joined together in long chains.

Fats, on the other hand, are either saturated or unsaturated. The two types of unsaturated fats are either monounsaturated or polyunsaturated. All of this terminology can be somewhat overwhelming, but definitely worth familiarizing yourself with and quite helpful when reading labels for nutritional information.

I personally think of saturated fats as the really bad, black hat wearing guys because they tend to raise your total blood cholesterol level. Also, saturated fat is solid at room temperature, so you can imagine what it does once it settles on your thighs and stomach. In actuality, there is some truth to the somewhat humorous television commercials showing women walking around with gigantic sticky buns taped to their thighs and men with donuts as spare tires encircling their waists. I can certainly relate to those commercials and try to keep them in mind when I am tempted by a Krispy Crème donut or some other empty calorie snack on a weak day.

The average American diet is extremely high in saturated fats, which are a leading cause of cardiovascular disease. Red meat and some dairy products, such as ice cream, and cheese, are full of saturated fat. Everyone should be aware of the link between diets high in saturated fat and the incidence of certain types of cancer, most notably colon, breast, and prostate cancers.

A very important fact to consider when you are trying to lose excess body fat is that there are four calories in one gram of carbohydrates and four calories in one gram of protein, but there are nine calories in the same amount (one gram) of fat. In other words, fat contains over twice the amount of calories as does an equal amount of carbohydrates or protein. What does this mean to you? To put it simply, cut the fat and you automatically cut your total caloric intake.

As if all of this talk about fats weren't confusing enough, I would be remiss if I didn't discuss the latest term to make its way into headlines and onto the packages of some of our favorite products in the grocery store. Trans fatty acids or TFA's (often simply called trans fats) are the subject of much interest in recent years because some experts believe that they may be just as bad, if not worse, for your health than saturated fats. Unlike other fats, trans fats are neither required nor beneficial for health.

These little villains of the fat underworld are actually a type of unsaturated fat that is industrially created as a side effect of hydrogenation of plant oils. The hydrogenation process developed in the early nineteen hundreds and was first commercialized as the best seller Crisco in 1911. The end effect of hydrogenation is to add hydrogen atoms to unsaturated fats, making them more saturated. These more saturated fats have a higher melting point and a reduced tendency for oxidation, resulting in a longer shelf-life.

The hydrogenation process gives liquid fats the look and texture of a naturally hard fat such as butter. TFA's, in quantities normally consumed by most Americans, actually raise total blood cholesterol and LDL (bad) cholesterol in much the same way that saturated fats do. Large amounts of Trans fatty acids also may lower levels of HDL's (the good guys), increasing the risk of heart disease. Fortunately, as a result of closer scrutiny by health conscious individuals and researchers, many companies are voluntarily removing trans fats from their products, or establishing trans-free product lines.

TFA's are found in a variety of processed foods, including margarine, cookies, biscuits, and cakes. Fried fast foods such as doughnuts and French fries also contain high levels of trans fatty acids.

There is still a great deal of ongoing research on the subject of TFA's but a good rule of thumb is to avoid foods that contain partially hydrogenated vegetable oil and limit your intake of the above mentioned food products and start reading labels. Do not let a trans fat free label on a product fool you into thinking that it is free of saturated fat, however.

If you are not already doing so, it is a good idea to make it a point to start reading labels. Being aware of exactly what you are eating is much easier now that the nutrition facts are printed on food packages. Ingredients are labeled in descending order of predominance, meaning that the first ingredient listed is what the product has the most of, and so on.

Do not let words such as all natural or lite trick you, or be misled by terms such as 50 percent less fat. Ask yourself, "Less fat than what? The competition's highest fat version containing twenty-six grams of fat?" Also, remember that the fact that something is fat free does not necessarily mean it is good for you, or that you can eat as much as you want.

Be aware that not all products listing pure vegetable oil as an ingredient are low in saturated fat. Two types of vegetable oil; palm kernel and coconut oil (the tropical oils) are even higher in saturated fat than butter. Watch for these specifically on food labels. Another good rule of thumb is this: if something contains lard, do not eat it. Do not forget to read your labels specifically for saturated fat grams. I try to stay away from any snack that contains more than two or three grams of saturated fat per serving.

In general, monounsaturated fats, such as olive oil and canola oil, are better for you than polyunsaturated fats because monounsaturated fats raise the good part of blood cholesterol (HDL's, also know as high density lipoproteins) without significantly raising the total blood cholesterol level. Polyunsaturated fats, such as safflower, sunflower, corn, and soybean oils, do not have this positive effect on HDLs but do tend to reduce your total blood cholesterol level.

Although they are often referred to as good and bad cholesterol, HDLs and LDLs (low density lipoproteins) are actually fat protein compounds, not actual types of cholesterol (the prefix lipo refers to fat). Their purpose is to transport cholesterol through the bloodstream.

To simplify things a little, I often think of HDLs as the good guys that carry cholesterol out of the arteries. LDLs are basically the bad guys that contribute to deadly coronary heart disease by clogging the arteries.

Contrary to popular opinion, not all cholesterol is bad. Cholesterol is made naturally by the body and is necessary for normal body functions, such as the manufacturing of hormones and vitamin D. The liver and other tissues produce all of the cholesterol that your body needs, however, so it really isn't necessary to obtain it from your dietary intake. For this reason, a severe reduction in dietary intake of cholesterol, except in infants, probably is not harmful.

Unlike fats, which are found in foods of both plant and animal origin, dietary cholesterol is found only in certain foods of animal origin. Cholesterol is not found in foods of plant origin. While grocery shopping, I have recently noticed that certain foods of plant origin that have always been naturally cholesterol free (such as peanut butter) are now plastered with cholesterol free labels as if it were an astounding new breakthrough.

The richest source of cholesterol in foods is egg yolk. In fact, the yolk of one large egg contains close to the three hundred milligrams daily limit of cholesterol recommended by the American Heart Association. Red meats, organ meats, and dairy products such as cheese, butter, whole milk, and ice cream are also high in cholesterol.

The National Cholesterol Education Program considers a total blood cholesterol level of less than two hundred milligrams per deciliter desirable. The cholesterol that is manufactured by your body and also the cholesterol that is absorbed from the food you eat, is carried in the blood so that it can be used by all the different parts of the body, including muscle, the nervous system, and the heart.

When the cells of the body cannot absorb any more cholesterol, the excess begins to accumulate in the walls of the blood vessels. Over time, the build-up of plaque narrows the walls, which restricts the flow of blood and can eventually lead to heart attack and stroke.

You have probably heard about the benefits of eating certain types of fish that contain omega-3 fatty acids. The oils of some fish are just one of the sources of this special polyunsaturated fat, which is thought to have a preventive effect on heart disease. By increasing the time it takes the blood to clot, fish oil may reduce the chances of a blood clot in the heart blocking an artery and causing a heart attack.

Omega-3 fatty acids also may prevent blood cells from sticking to the insides of the blood vessels, which, in time, can build up and cause restriction of the blood flow. Cold-water fish such as mackerel, salmon, tuna, sardines, and herring are excellent sources of omega-3 fatty acids. Eating these types of fish is generally preferable to taking fish oil capsules. I am always cautious about eating too much fish, however, because of possible high mercury content. Flaxseed oil, canola oil, walnuts, and almonds are also good sources of omega-3 fatty acids.

A major source of cholesterol in the diets of many American children, teenagers, and adults comes from eating at fast food chains, which spend an average of nearly one billion dollars a year in television advertising alone. Although some fast food restaurants are beginning to offer somewhat healthier choices, most fast foods are still low in nutrients and fiber, and extremely high in fat and sodium.

Many people mistakenly believe that they are eating healthily when they order chicken or fish at fast food restaurants. What they may not be aware of, however, is that if the item is fried, it can still derive more than half of its calories from fat. While some dietary fat is necessary for optimal health, your body was not designed to live on Double Whoppers with cheese, containing 935 calories and sixty-one grams of fat.

I believe that our society's reliance on fast food is partially responsible for the fact that almost everyone knows a person who has died of heart disease at an early age. When that person is a friend or family member, the statistics and information about heart disease hit a little closer to home.

I once spent a physically and emotionally challenging month driving back and forth to a hospital in another part of the state to visit a close relative who underwent extensive heart surgery. Like many people his age (at the time he was in his late sixties) he grew up eating high quantities of red meat, butter, cheese, ice cream, and other foods high in saturated fat. Exercise had been a low priority during this loved one's life, and stress prevention and reduction were unheard of in his younger days.

Over the years, his condition had progressed slowly, silently clogging his arteries with no outward signs until a week before he was hospitalized. Observing him and other heart patients suffering in the intensive care unit, hooked up to a maze of wires and tubes, and sympathizing with the grief stricken friends and family of other patients who did not fare as well, was saddening to say the least.

Something positive did come out of the experience, however. He survived the ordeal and changed his lifestyle and I became even more determined to share the information I have gathered through the years about making necessary lifestyle changes to increase the odds of living a long, healthy life.

Maintaining a low level of saturated dietary fat is one of the few rules on which most nutrition experts seem to agree. Who knows how many lives could be saved simply by making the decision to cut back on or eliminate red meat and fast food in one's diet? I cannot overemphasize how important it is to be aware of the sources of your dietary fat.

Although reducing fat can save lives, it is important to remember that good nutrition, like good health, is not simply the absence of something. It is also the presence or addition of something positive, such as antioxidant rich vegetables, fruits, whole grains, and legumes. Maintaining a proper level of dietary fat is just one crucial piece of the puzzle. In order to see the whole picture, you need to work with all of the pieces.

As I pointed out earlier, stress is also a major contributing factor to heart disease, as is lack of exercise. A person who maintains a low fat diet, yet never exercises, and leads a stressful life can still be susceptible to heart disease. By practicing what you have learned from using the Pura Vida stepping stones, and respecting and understanding the unity of the mind, body, and spirit, you can reduce your risk of killer heart disease and other life threatening conditions.

Your health and well-being are affected by many integrally related factors. During my life, I have come to believe that negative emotions such as anger and hostility can be just as harmful as eating bacon for breakfast every morning, and that if everyone spent more time meditating or praying, laughing, and loving, there would be fewer cardiovascular related deaths and less disease in the world.

Without a doubt, the average American diet is extremely high in fat and many people make the wrong nutritional decisions simply because they are not well informed. For this reason, I will further discuss dietary fat in upcoming chapters in order to share what I have discovered thus far in my own quest for the truth.

I urge you to extract whatever information you find helpful along your own daily journey, all the while maintaining your steady pure momentum, experimenting with, and applying what you have learned along the way. Your cumulative knowledge and experience will serve to strengthen the foundation of your current health belief system as you, too, discover your own truth—one step at a time.

Reflective Interlude

Before we delve further into the exciting, yet practical and fact filled areas of nutrition and exercise, perhaps now is a good time to slow down, reflect upon, and review your journey thus far. Take a little time to breathe deeply, recharge your batteries, swing from the vines, dip your feet in the pools of a soothing waterfall, and give yourself credit where it is due.

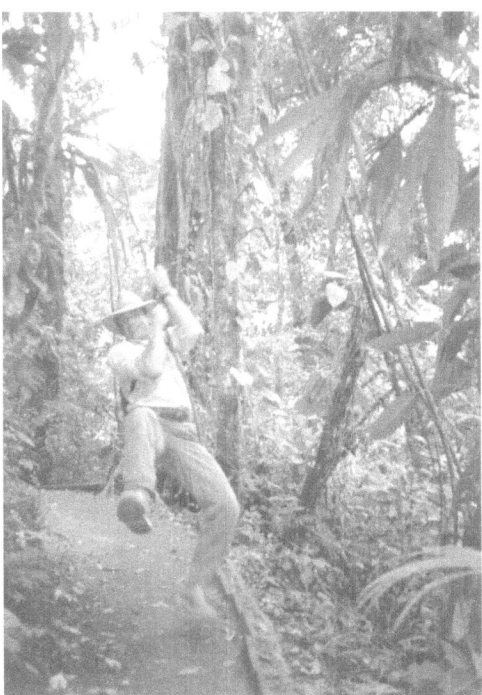

Ask yourself if you are applying what you have learned from the Pura Vida stepping stones on a daily basis or simply plunging forward into the next chapter of your life without fully living in this moment. When you realize that life is a continuous succession of present moments, and not a frenetic race, it is much easier to break the habits of hurrying and worrying about the future, or dwelling on the past.

In the following chapters, you will learn a great deal of practical information that can help change the direction of your life and provide you with unlimited, boundless energy. Before you proceed, however, it is important that you have created a solid foundation by taking full advantage of the Pura Vida Stepping Stones.

Living in today's sometimes frenetically paced world of traffic jams, over scheduling, and overdevelopment, it is easy to lose your connection with the earth and all of the healthy gifts that nature has to offer.

Tony, our friend and guide to the hidden wonders of Costa Rica, shared an interesting story with us that reinforced our belief in the importance of spending quality time in nature on a regular basis. Tony was raised in the rolling green countryside of Texas and could certainly be described as a nature boy. When he was in his first year of college, he won a prestigious art competition. His award included a two week stay in New York City, which allowed him to study at some of the finest museums the world has to offer.

Like many people accustomed to small town living, Tony's initial response to the Big Apple was one of awe, excitement, and what I think of as sensory overload or over stimulation. Tony quickly found that he was unable to sleep well and that despite the powerful creative and intellectual stimulation he was experiencing, his health and energy level were rapidly deteriorating.

As he told us his story, we could easily picture him striding through the busy, clamoring streets of the city with his long, braided ponytail swinging on top of his weathered leather backpack. As his appetite, energy level, and strength diminished, Tony considered returning to his country home ahead of schedule. He changed his mind, however, when he acted on an impulse and most likely surprised a few of even the most world-weary city dwellers who were people-watching while dining in a fine outdoor restaurant on Park Avenue.

As Tony's well-traveled hiking boots relentlessly pounded the pavement, he suddenly realized that his feet had touched nothing but concrete, tile, bricks, and carpet since he had left his peaceful home. It was the dead of winter, there were no leaves on the trees, and he had not seen the sun for ten days. At that moment, Tony spotted a large planter filled with fresh, rich brown soil outside of an upscale Manhattan restaurant.

We could barely contain our laughter as Tony continued to tell us the rest of his story. Unable to control himself, he dug his brightly colored, paint stained hands into the dark, loamy soil of the planter, scooping and sifting the dirt until someone from the hotel began to approach him. According to Tony, he immediately felt more energetic and calm and quickly realized that the reason he had been feeling so unhealthy was that he had totally lost his connection with the earth.

He then decided to skip his classes for the rest of the afternoon and seek out the infamous Central Park. There he spent the remainder of the day joyfully exploring the lovely paths and gardens, fantastically gnarled old trees, and interesting nooks and crannies of this little bit of heaven surrounded by the imposing walls of the concrete canyon.

As a country girl at heart, I can relate to Tony's amusing story. Since childhood, I have always felt strongly about spending quality time in nature, and connecting with the earth. Naturally, the Pure Life trailblazers also felt so strongly about this concept that they made this principle an important stepping stone along the Pura Vida pathway.

Stepping Stone # 10: *Spend as much quality time in Nature as possible, connecting with your life force and breathing deeply.*

I have found that when I am in tune with nature, I am more in tune with my spiritual core, and also with my physical body and busy mind. When you spend time appreciating the glorious colors of the rising and setting sun, or listening to the wind whispering through the trees, you will also experience more meaningful real moments in your everyday life.

The more that we all recharge our batteries by spending time in nature, the more open we are to unexpected, meaningful coincidences and experiences which help point us in the right direction and maintain our positive, pure momentum.

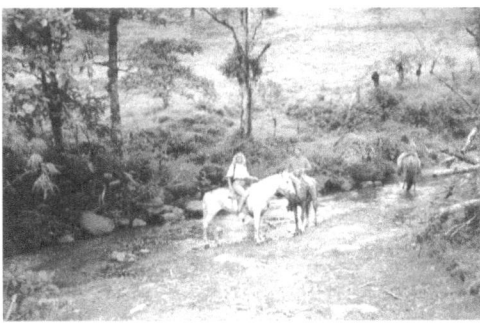

As you continue to explore the mysterious, ever changing world along your unique path, make it a high priority to spend time in natural settings, and continue to be aware of the signs and coincidences in your everyday life. As you do so, take time to listen to your innate wisdom before making health related decisions.

Never lose sight of the fact that you are the creator of your own lifestyle or way of living, and that a harmonious balance of your mind, body, and soul is the key not only to optimal health and free flowing, pure energy, but also to peace, joy, and success. Regardless of the challenges and obstacles you may be currently facing, your life is a miraculous gift—a unique, meaningful adventure that is continuously progressing and unfolding, one step at a time. You are not the same person that you were yesterday or that you will be tomorrow.

When you begin assimilating the positive information that you have accumulated into your daily lifestyle, you will change even more rapidly and become even more closely connected to the comforting pulse of the earth, and to your own powerful inner energy and strength.

Use this interlude to reflect on how far you have come, strengthen your resolve to continue making healthy choices, and prepare for the next exhilarating chapter of your Pure Life Odyssey. No hurries, no worries!

The Transition Stage

If you are at the point along your path where you are ready to permanently change unhealthy eating habits but have previously had difficulty breaking years of conditioning, I would like to recommend the following tips for what I like to call the transition stage. During the transition stage, you can begin gradually changing your eating habits by reducing fat, processed sugar, salt, and chemical additives while replacing unhealthy favorites with more nutritious substitutes.

If you have already passed through this stage, congratulations. You have discovered that proper nutrition truly is an essential component of your personal voyage of pure health with its own unique benefits and rewards.

As you read the following information, please keep in mind that much of this text was written during the period that I saw several friends and loved ones losing their lives to cardiovascular disease, so there is considerable emphasis on dietary fat.

If you have always eaten a traditional fat filled diet, but are ready to make some changes, you do not have to go cold turkey in order to reduce your dietary fat intake. You can gradually wean yourself from eating excessive amounts of dietary fat, if you wish. For example, you can begin by switching from whole milk, which is 3.5% fat by weight, to 2% milk. (If you have always thought that 2% milk is low in fat, consider this: 33% of its calories come from fat. The 2% refers only to its fat content by weight).

After your taste buds have had time to adjust to 2% milk, you may choose to drop down to 1%, then eventually to skim milk. After you have made the transition to skim, take a sip of whole milk. You may be surprised by how heavy and thick it now seems, and you may even think, "How did I ever drink that?" It can take up to three months for your taste buds to adapt to dietary fat changes, so allow sufficient time for the transition to take place.

It is much easier to give up the fatty foods that you may currently crave when you have a replacement for them. You may find it more effective to replace your high fat food items a little at a time. On your next trip to the grocery store, make it a point to exchange at least one item for a replacement low fat item. Continue until you have replaced all the high fat foods in your pantry and refrigerator.

When you are ready, you may want to start exchanging lower fat items with fat free versions.

Be careful, however, not to get too comfortable at this point in the transition stage. Do not fool yourself by assuming that simply because your kitchen is full of low fat, processed food products that you are eating as well as you possibly can. Fat free Devil's food cookies and low fat fudge brownies are not health promoting foods, no matter how attractively they are marketed.

Depending on the overall nutritional content, low fat or fat free products are not necessarily the end result of your nutritional journey. In many cases, they are simply temporary crutches that help you to permanently say goodbye to an unhealthy, high fat diet.

In some cases, such as switching from whole to skim milk, the main nutritional difference is a reduced fat content and the product does not lose its nutritional value. In other products, however, more sugar or salt are added to low fat or fat free food products than the original high fat version. This is why that during this stage, it is important to keep reading your labels, not only for fat content, but also for sodium, sugars, additives, and preservatives.

Compare different brands and manufacturers. Spend a little time in the health food aisle of your grocery store, or better yet, in a health food store. Instead of wasting time trying to make sense of the latest fad diet book, simply be completely honest with yourself about the types and amounts of foods that make up the majority of your diet. Concentrate on what you instinctively know are your weak areas.

Rather than trying to follow a complicated diet plan or program that does not work in real life, strengthen your resolve to give up the empty calorie foods, binges, or fast foods that may be at the root of your unhealthy eating habits.

If you have never stepped foot in your local health food store, but recognize many of the faces at your favorite fast food drive up window, it is time to be adventurous and veer off of your familiar path, or in this case, comfortable rut.

Health food stores are not the mystical, mysterious, or even strange places that some people may have perceived them to be in the past. Not everyone who shops at health food stores wears tie-dye clothing and smells of incense (not that there is anything wrong with that). Although some health food stores are notoriously expensive, we have found a few close to our home that are reasonably priced and offer a good selection of organic produce and products.

Today, it is much easier to find organic products that are also low in fat than it was a few years ago. Remember to read your labels for fat content, even in the health food store. It is usually less expensive to buy foods such as grains and legumes in bulk.

I like experimenting with new foods and have actually come to enjoy the taste of foods such as organic rice milk and lentil soup. Frozen organic veggie burgers and soy dogs taste much better than they sound and only take a few minutes to prepare.

I do not believe, however, that it is necessary to spend your whole paycheck at the health food store in order to provide your body with quality fuel for your journey. With a little research, comparison-shopping, and experimentation, however, you can increase the quality and amount of pure energy foods in your diet by shopping at these alternative markets more often.

I also urge you to further explore different trails along your new path by experimenting with recipes from the multitude of healthy cookbooks that are currently available. Ask friends and family about their timesaving, fat-reducing secrets. The amount of valuable, practical information that you can obtain by steering the conversation in the right direction may surprise you. Encourage your friends and family to join you on your new adventure—the more the merrier.

While continuing your exploration and research, you may choose to take advantage of the toll free numbers listed on most products. A few years ago, I discovered some very interesting facts about fat and food labeling by making a few simple phone calls to satisfy my own curiosity.

It all began when I was reading labels in the cooking oil aisle at the grocery store. I discovered that every type of oil I picked up had fourteen grams of fat per tablespoon. While looking at the label of the fat free cooking spray that I sometimes use, I noticed that it contains safflower oil. I wondered how it could be classified as fat free since it contained oil.

One day, out of curiosity, I called the toll free number listed on the can and found that the answer was in the serving size. For this product, one serving was considered as one-third of a second of spray, which in my experience does not cover a very large surface.

Another phone call, this time to the F.D.A., verified that if a product contains less than .05 gram of fat per serving, which is considered a trivial amount, it can be labeled as fat free. In actuality, in the 744 servings contained in this one can, there was a total of approximately 185 grams of fat.

What this little lesson taught me was this; for manufacturers to be able to label their products fat free, they may reduce the serving size to ensure that it stays below the F.D.A.'s parameters—yet another reason to pay special attention to serving sizes while reading labels.

I also learned that the words high, rich in, or an excellent source of, in connection with any nutrient mean that the product must contain at least 20% of the recommended daily value for that nutrient per serving. To be labeled as a good source of a certain nutrient, one serving must contain 10–19% of the daily value for that particular nutrient. Also, the words 95% fat free on a label means that the food contains five grams or less of fat per one hundred grams of the food.

Although reducing dietary fat is crucial in the fight against cardiovascular disease and obesity, it is important to be aware that many low fat and fat free foods still contain high levels of simple sugars and salt. Remember, fat free does not mean calorie free, and is not always synonymous with guilt free.

As you raise your level of nutritional awareness by educating yourself, you too will discover some surprising facts about your old favorite foods. For example:

- A seven ounce platter of nachos with twelve ounces of cheddar cheese contains 2,498 calories and 174.5 grams of fat.

- Ten potato skins sprinkled with cheddar cheese contain 60.5 grams of fat and 1,034 calories.

- A bag of natural potato chips gets 60 percent of its calories from fat.

As you venture along your new, ever changing nutritional path, gaining energizing momentum by researching, substituting, and experimenting, you may discover a challenging spot in the form of one of America's favorite pastimes—eating out.

Making the right nutritional decisions when you are eating out at a restaurant takes some practical knowledge and quite a bit of healthy discipline. One trick that I have found helpful is to eat a small piece of fruit or other healthy snack before I leave the house. That way, your stomach is not growling by the time your food arrives, and dessert is not quite so tempting. Also, do not be afraid to ask the waiter for low fat suggestions. Most restaurants are finally starting to see the lite and offer more heart smart choices.

When ordering from a menu, avoid anything with the dirty word fried. You are usually better off with something that is broiled, baked, roasted, or grilled. Some other no-no's are gravy, cheese, creamed, parmigiana, white sauce, crispy, au gratin, batter dipped, breaded, and flaky. Chicken and fish are usually a better choice than beef. Make sure that they are skinless and not fried, however.

When ordering pasta, veer away from the creamy white sauces such as fettucine alfredo, which can have more than sixty grams of fat and one thousand calories in a three cup serving. Stick to the red marinara type sauces. Ask your server to hold or go light on the cheese. Again, pay special attention to serving sizes.

When eaten in moderation, bread (especially if it is a dark, hearty whole grain) is not as fattening as you may think. It is the amount that you eat and the butter you put on it that can be your downfall. Be aware that soup and salad is not always a low calorie or low fat choice, especially if the soup is a fat-filled, creamy bisque or chowder and if the salad is drenched in heavy, oily dressing.

Do not be afraid to ask if the restaurant offers any low fat or fat free dressings. Always ask for the salad dressing on the side and use it sparingly, or try a little virgin olive oil and vinegar or light vinegarette dressing. Be aware that bacon bits, avocado, sunflower seeds, and cheese are high in fat.

Regardless of what your mother always told you about the starving children in Africa, you do not always have to be a member of the clean plate club. Tonight's take-home may be tomorrow's quick and easy lunch.

Something that I have learned from personal experience over the years is that it is extremely important to avoid eating too much food in the evening. Many people with weight problems eat the majority of their calories after 5:00 PM, when their bodies need the energy the least. I highly recommend eating the bulk of your calories earlier in the day. That way, they are more likely to be used as pure energy rather than stored as excess bodyfat. Remember this fact the next time you are staring into the refrigerator wondering what to have for a late night snack.

Also, remember that your body functions most efficiently when you spread your calories throughout the day. By eating many, mini-meals, you will keep your blood sugar at a more consistent level and positively affect your metabolic rate.

Do not wait until you are shaky and weak to eat. Usually, by the time you get to this point, you are more concerned with what you can eat the quickest, not with what choice has the most nutritional value. Plan ahead and supply your body with quality fuel for your high quality, high energy, Pura Vida lifestyle.

Regardless of exactly where you are on your nutritional path, I hope that you are taking time to practice what you have learned on a daily basis and incorporating the changes into your changing lifestyle. Wherever you are, take time to enjoy the view, gaze at the stars, and step back a little in order to see the whole picture. Always keeps in mind that listening to your inner voice and nourishing your soul are just as important as nourishing your body with high quality food.

Dietary Fat Reduction Tips

In this chapter, you'll find some quick and easy tips that will help you reduce dietary fat and replace some of your old unhealthy favorites, as you continue further through the transition stage.

Since an increasingly high percentage of our country's population is both overweight and at risk for heart attack and stroke, the following information was written with these facts in mind. Contrary to what the billion dollar pharmaceutical advertising industry would have us believe, taking drugs such as Lipitor and Zocor for the rest of your life is not always the smartest solution to lowering your cholesterol and decreasing your odds of dying from cardiovascular disease.

Of course, many lives have been saved by using these drugs once the problem is out of control, but the answer lies in prevention and in permanently changing your overall lifestyle while being consciously aware of what you eat on a daily basis.

I apologize for the fact that my recipes are somewhat lacking in the measurement department, but I am strictly a pinch of this, a dash of that cook, constantly experimenting, rarely making a dish the same way twice.

If you have not already begun doing so, try replacing high fat ingredients with healthier alternatives in your recipes. You can substitute applesauce for butter and margarine, eliminate egg yolks, or use low fat yogurt instead of mayonnaise in your recipes and meals.

Simply by substituting applesauce for butter in your muffins, breads, and cakes, you can save more than nine hundred calories and one hundred grams of fat for each one-half cup of applesauce you use. In recipes that call for oil, try using half applesauce and half low fat buttermilk for similar fat and calorie saving benefits.

You can also substitute ground turkey for hamburger in your recipes. Try to find white meat ground turkey or see if the butcher can grind it for you. It costs a little more, but contains much less fat than dark turkey meat.

As a substitute for traditional meatloaf, try making turkey meatloaf with salsa and fresh vegetables. Replace ground beef with ground white turkey meat; add plenty of salsa, fresh tomatoes, or tomato sauce, one or two egg whites, a few crushed whole wheat crackers, plenty of seasoning, onions, garlic, green peppers, mushrooms, tomatoes, corn—whatever you like. Kids even like turkey meatloaf and it makes great sandwiches the next day.

If you have tried reduced fat cheese once or twice but just could not tolerate the taste, you may want to give it another chance by gradually sneaking it into salads, sandwiches, and omelets during the transition stage.

I have always liked the taste of real cheese, but after a few months using the healthier lower fat alternative, I hardly noticed the difference. Quite honestly, however, I never could quite adjust to the taste of fat free cheese, but adapted fairly quickly to low fat cheese. Eventually, I found that simply leaving cheese out of recipes and sandwiches was not as difficult as I thought it would be.

As a healthy alternative to saturated fat filled, fast food pizza, try making vegetarian pizza. Add sliced, fresh tomatoes, green peppers, onions, mushrooms, garlic, spinach, and hot peppers if you like. They are all delicious and good for you, as is a hearty tomato sauce. You may want to use a small amount of mozzarella or reduced fat cheese. Just say no to the sausage, pepperoni, and layers of high fat cheese, however. If you like meat on your pizza, experiment with shrimp or low fat ham or turkey.

I sometimes use fat free, low sodium chicken broth as a base for cooking soups and main dishes. Also, chicken baked in low sodium, fat free cream of mushroom soup is a very tasty alternative to fried chicken. Serve with brown rice for extra energy boosting complex carbohydrates. When choosing any canned goods, including soups and broths, always remember to check the label for high sodium levels.

If you must use oil when you cook, spray your pans with a small amount of non-fat cooking spray or use a little olive or canola oil (the good, monounsaturated type fats), also available in sprays. Try adding a little water when baking chicken, turkey, or fish. Not only will occasionally adding small amounts of water prevent sticking but it can actually make meat more tender. I have also found that baking in folded aluminum foil helps keep meat tender and juicy and makes oil less necessary.

I like to experiment with different herbs and natural seasonings, often using fresh herbs from our garden, which add flavor to everything we cook. Using plenty of natural herbs and seasonings made it easier for us to cut back on salt and makes low fat foods taste a little more zesty and exciting. Lemon juice and salsa are also tasty, fat free seasonings that enhance the flavor of food, but are very often overlooked. Try adding plenty of fresh squeezed lemon juice to salads and fish recipes.

Do not ruin nutritious foods like whole grain pasta, potatoes, and salad, by smothering them with heavy sauces, butter, and dressings. Baked potatoes are rich in complex carbohydrates and free of fat and cholesterol, if you do not drown them in butter and sour cream. They are also high in fiber, vitamin C, potassium, iron, and B vitamins. Try topping them with low fat or fat free sour cream, steamed broccoli, low fat cheeses, low fat or fat free cottage cheese, black beans, or salsa. The skin of baked potatoes is also a great source of dietary fiber.

As we found in Costa Rica, it is a good idea to keep a box or two of nonfat dry milk in the cupboard for times when you run out of skim milk. Add a little vanilla extract, and you have a tasty, fat-free backup.

I have found that one of the most practical ways to increase our consumption of fresh vegetables is to always have some vegetable soup or stew going. I call my zesty soups Love Soup because you can practically taste the love that goes into preparing fresh, hearty hot soup. A big pot of soup is also great for feeding company and for busy people who don't always have the luxury of eating at specific times.

You may have heard of the fat burning cabbage soup recipes going around the rapid weight loss centers. As you probably suspected, there is not a magical ingredient in cabbage that makes you lose weight, but having something hot and healthy around to eat when you are hungry does decrease the chances that you will reach for something quick and fattening. Also, when you satisfy your nutritional needs with something such as fresh vegetable soup, you will find that you are less likely to crave junk food.

Crock-pots can be a lifesaver. I almost always have something simmering in mine. Fill yours full of fresh (preferably organic) vegetables, tomato sauce, seasoning, beans, lean chicken, and other healthy stuff. What I like best about it is that you can turn the crock pot on low, go to work or the gym, and you do not have to worry about what to make for dinner when you get home. Soups made with vegetable and potatoes have a tendency to get a little mushy when cooked too long in a crock pot. I usually transfer mine to another container or cooking pot after the first meal.

Bean soup is just one of my many crock-pot staples and an excellent source of quality protein. Clean and soak whole dried beans (the more variety the better), add plenty of water and seasonings, and cook on low. You may also want to add carrots, celery, fresh herbs, and onions.

Crock-pots are also great for cooking marinara and spaghetti sauces. Try making a nice, homemade marina sauce with lots of salt free seasonings to use over pasta, and save the rest of the sauce for making a pizza or to use in a healthy soup.

You can also make a tasty, hearty chili that I like to call White Chicken Chili. Simply combine small pieces of lean white chicken or turkey breast, your favorite beans, a can of fat free chili, salsa, fresh tomatoes or organic diced tomatoes, peppers, onions, garlic, herbs, and seasonings, and let cook in your trusty crock pot until done. You may need to experiment with the amount of tomato sauce needed for the consistency that you desire. Make sure that the chicken is thoroughly cooked, as well.

If you prefer to cook on the stovetop, lightly spray your cooking pot with a low fat or fat free spray such as canola or olive oil and brown the chicken, peppers, onions, and garlic first. Then add the additional ingredients and let them cook at a low heat. I usually add the beans last so that they do not become overly soft. Be creative! It is easier than you might think.

Perhaps the best tip that I have to offer is the simplest. If you do not already have one, buy a vegetable steamer and use it. Leave it out on your countertop if you need a reminder. Steaming not only retains vital nutrients but also enhances flavor. It really does not take long to steam veggies, and they add a nice, wholesome, homemade touch to any meal.

We got hooked on black beans and rice, a.k.a. *arroz y frijoles*, while we were in Costa Rica. The Ticos even eat this satisfying dish for breakfast. Beans and brown rice are an excellent source of complete protein and complex carbohydrates, and are quick, easy, and inexpensive to make. We sometimes eat black beans and rice three or four times a week, and have found that this simple meal can avert dietary disaster, especially at times when our refrigerator is empty and we are tempted to order in or eat out.

Here is the bachelor-approved recipe for Dr. Suzy's Super Easy *Arroz y Frijoles*. When shopping for black beans, look for the brand with the least amount of fat and salt. Put the beans in a microwave safe container and heat them. Then, boil one bag of instant, boil-in-bag brown rice. Mix the beans and rice together and season with herbal seasonings instead of salt. This makes enough for two or three people.

Beans and rice are also good with chicken, shrimp, or vegetables. We like peas in ours. Who says there is no such thing as healthy fast food? It doesn't get any easier than that. Beans and rice are even better for you when prepared with unprocessed organic brown rice and fresh dried beans because they contain more of their original nutrients. A good timesaving option is to cook a big batch of whole grain, brown rice and dried beans, and then freeze smaller portions for later use.

We love tacos, but most taco shells are loaded with fat, so we make Guilt Free Chicken Fajitas as a delicious alternative. Begin by cooking the chicken without adding oil and use skinless, boneless white meat, cut into long strips. Fire up the grill or broiler, or cook stovetop with a small amount of fat free canola or olive oil spray. Season the chicken with garlic, salsa, pepper, and herbal seasonings.

Wrap the chicken in a fat free or low fat tortilla shell, along with chopped tomatoes, green peppers, onions and spinach or lettuce. You can add fat free vegetarian refried beans, as well. Top with salsa, low fat or fat-free sour cream or reduced fat cheese, but hold the guacamole. The end result is messy but very tasty and well worth the effort. Save the leftovers for making a nutritious, protein rich egg white omelet the next morning.

You may also want to try making nutrient filled sweet potato wedges instead of traditional greasy French fries. Hopefully, your kids will like this one too. Clean two or three sweet potatoes, and cut in wedges like French fries. Place on a cookie sheet and lightly cover with fat free olive or canola oil cooking spray. Cook at 350°, turning once until both sides are slightly crispy. Sweet potatoes are loaded with vitamins and minerals, so experiment with different ways of cooking them.

Another staple in our pantry is protein rich canned tuna in spring water. We especially like white albacore tuna with a little low fat ranch dressing, plenty of dill and other fresh herbs, a little celery, chopped egg white, fresh lemon juice, and sometimes a very small amount of chopped pickle. Be sure to only buy tuna that is packed in water, not fat filled oil.

Hot air or microwave popcorn (minus the butter) is a great, quick snack food that is full of fiber and can help curb your appetite. Try putting a little chili powder or nonfat Parmesan cheese on popcorn for a different tasting snack.

As frequent moviegoers, we know first hand how tempting it is to pass up the tantalizing smell of dangerously fattening theater popcorn. Even without the butter, however, a large bucket of movie theater popcorn that has been popped in coconut oil may contain the equivalent of three days allotment of saturated fat.

The solution? I must confess that we sometimes sneak our own low fat snacks into the movies. Fat free pretzels and low fat microwave popcorn are just a few of the snacks that are easily smuggled in a backpack or large purse. We sometimes bring a container of water, as well.

For a healthy, quick dessert loaded with potassium, try making a frozen *Banana con Leche* (banana with milk). Bananas are easily digested and contain potassium and vitamins A, B-complex, and C. Rather than letting your bananas go bad when they start becoming a little too brown, peel them and put them in the freezer in a Ziploc bag.

When you are ready for a cold, sweet treat, put three or four of the frozen bananas in the blender with some skim or rice milk and a little vanilla extract or even some yogurt or protein powder. This tasty treat is much more satisfying and better for you than a saturated fat filled milkshake. We got hooked on these while frequenting a very cool health food restaurant called *El Sano Banana* (the healthy banana) in Montezuma, Costa Rica. Backpackers and expatriates from all over the world gathered here in the evening sipping *banana con leches* and watching nightly open air movies shown on a big screen in the middle of the jungle.

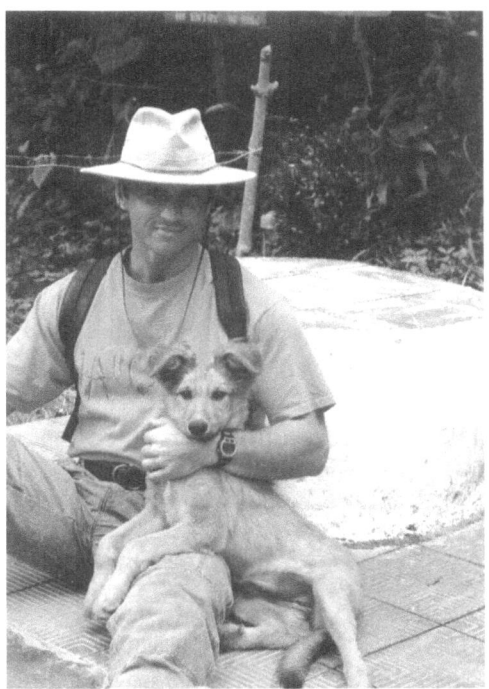

Experiment with blending other frozen fruits such as strawberries, kiwis, blackberries, peaches, and melons. With some creativity, you may find a new favorite healthy dessert without all the added sugars, fat, and chemicals. Frozen grapes are another pleasant hot weather treat. We especially like them at the beach on a sizzling summer day.

We frequently use a hand blender to make protein drinks, especially on days when we have had a particularly strenuous workout. We usually use powdered egg white protein, but sometimes make shakes with spirulina based protein powder from the health food store.

You can add fat free yogurt, wheat germ, and just about any combination of juices and fruits for a never-ending variety of healthy protein drinks at any time of day. A removable detachment on the hand blender makes clean up quick and easy.

Instead of hiding our fruits and vegetables in some dark, lonely spot in the back of the refrigerator, I make it a point to bring them to the front or put them out in a bowl. Keeping them in sight reminds us to eat them. We also cut up celery, carrots, cauliflower, and broccoli and store in the refrigerator in Ziploc bags for a quick snack. They're also great for snacking in the car or away from home when already prepared to eat.

One of our favorite toppings, wheat germ, truly is a health food. A one-fourth cup serving of wheat germ supplies more than half of your daily magnesium, folic acid, iron, and zinc, and is loaded with vitamin E.

For added calcium and magnesium, we sometimes sprinkle wheat germ on non fat yogurt and frozen yogurt. We usually choose plain yogurt and add fresh fruit and vanilla, because the sugar content of commercial fruited yogurts is rather high. I also love the nutty taste of heart healthy flaxseed and try to keep it handy in the fridge to sprinkle in various recipes or over cereal.

Because eating breakfast kicks in your metabolism earlier in the day and supplies you with much needed energy, breakfast really is your most important meal. Luckily, breakfast does not have to be boring. There are many healthy options to choose from, including fresh fruit, juice, egg white omelets, whole grain cereals, oatmeal, and low fat bran muffins.

Omelets made with egg whites are an excellent source of protein any time of the day. Experiment with different seasonings and add fresh tomatoes, peppers, onions, broccoli, spinach, mushrooms, low fat cheese, or healthy leftovers. Serve the eggs with wheat toast or low fat bran or oat bagels and fat free cottage cheese on the side. Try using a little honey instead of cream cheese on your bagel.

Don't be afraid to mix it up a little. For a Spanish touch, try the lower fat version of traditional *Huevos Rancheros*. Cook egg whites or egg substitutes with whatever vegetables you like, add salsa and beans and roll in fat free tortillas. A quick alternative to greasy home fries is cubed potatoes cooked in a zip lock bag in the microwave. Simply sprinkle seasoning in the bag, shake it around, and cook until soft.

Whole grain cereal with skim milk can be a quick and nutritious energy booster any time of the day. Stay away from the refined, sugar coated varieties, however. Choose the high fiber, low sugar, whole grain types instead. Again, do not be fooled by words like all natural. Even healthy sounding granola can be full of sugar and extremely high in saturated fats such as palm and coconut oil. The only way to know for sure is to read the label.

Another breakfast favorite that we discovered in Costa Rica is buckwheat pancakes with bananas. Although we were never able to duplicate the delicious jam-like topping, which included some mysterious, soft, tasty bark, we have concocted our own recipe for Banana Buckwheats by simply following the buckwheat pancake box recipe and adding thinly sliced bananas to the batter before cooking. We lightly spray the pan with a fat free canola spray and use applesauce instead of oil and usually leave out the egg yolk.

As I mentioned earlier, Len and I frequently start the day with a bowl of uncooked, organic, old-fashioned oats and Grape Nuts with skim milk or rice milk. Top with a little honey, raisins, or sliced banana if you like. It tastes much better than it sounds. Try it at least once and see if you do not notice a difference in your energy level.

Remember, your health is a direct result of the decisions that you make on a daily basis. If you decide to have fresh corn on the cob, grilled fish, and a green salad for dinner tonight instead of greasy fast food, it will directly affect every other aspect of your life.

You will have more energy to turn the challenges that may be facing you into opportunities. Your body chemistry will produce a more positive and focused emotional state. Your digestive system will function more efficiently, causing fewer unpleasant side effects and symptoms. Put simply, in order to experience the life enhancing power and pure energy that come from taking care of yourself, you must provide your body with the proper fuel to run on.

Of course, you are not always going to make the right choices. None of us are perfect and no one would enjoy being around us if we were. What really matters is that you keep moving forward in the right direction, and that you do not lose sight of your everyday lifestyle goals.

You possess the ultimate gift—the freedom of choice—and you have chosen to be as healthy, happy, and strong as possible. It is entirely up to you to make sure that your daily nutritional decisions are in line with that choice. It is up to you to navigate your own passage through life, concentrating on your own requirements for personal growth and optimal health.

Your willingness to learn, grow, and make healthy choices will liberate new energy—energy which supports a new way of being. This transformational energy has a ripple effect on every other aspect of your life, so do not waste another second. Seize the moment!

Sodium Balance

There is a hidden substance in our foods that is at the center of much recent controversy. Whether or not excess dietary sodium is the potentially lethal substance that scientists once believed remains to be seen. Most experts do agree, however, that the average American consumes far more sodium than the body needs for proper functioning.

Table salt, also known as sodium chloride, is about 40 percent sodium by weight. The F.D.A. recommends that you consume 2,400 mg of sodium a day, which is roughly the amount in one teaspoon of salt. An adequate level of sodium is necessary for the body to function properly. Sodium is an essential part of a healthy diet and a severe deficiency of this mineral can cause death. Sodium occurs naturally in some foods and is best obtained naturally, not from the salt shaker habit or from processed foods.

Excessive sodium consumption is just one of the risk factors linked with high blood pressure. Many experts agree that certain people are sodium sensitive and, for them, too much salt can cause a sustained increase in blood pressure. There is currently some debate about exactly what percentage of the population is sensitive to the blood pressure elevating effects of sodium, and to what extent. Other factors, such as smoking, stress, improper nutrition, lack of exercise, and obesity, also enter prominently into the cardiovascular picture.

Sodium, along with potassium, regulates the body's acid balance and is necessary for proper functioning of nerves and muscles. Sodium and potassium are also crucial minerals in the exchange of cellular fluids, forming an amazing mechanism called the sodium potassium pump.

Maintaining the delicate balance between these two minerals is essential in bringing nutrients into the cells and pumping wastes out of them. When this balance is thrown off, usually by a buildup of sodium, excess fluids accumulate in the tissues, causing the body to retain water. For this reason, excessive sodium consumption can result in excessive water weight gain and fluid retention, commonly known as bloating.

Water retention can make blood pressure that is already high rise even higher. Furthermore, excessive sodium intake may also increase your chances of osteoporosis, since it causes your body to lose calcium. For these reasons, we decided to cut back on sodium years ago, mainly by breaking the saltshaker habit and by becoming more aware of the sodium content in our favorite foods.

Cutting down on your sodium intake is not as difficult as you might think. It may be hard for you to imagine eating foods without adding salt. Once you wean yourself, however, many of your old favorites often taste too salty, because the taste for salt is more of an acquired taste than that of sugar or fat.

Start watching labels for ingredients containing the word sodium, including sodium sulfate, or monosodium glutamate (MSG). Use garlic powder or onion powder instead of garlic salt or onion salt, and use low sodium broth instead of bouillon cubes. If you must have something to shake on your food, experiment with the salt substitutes for the transition stage.

Be aware that a no salt added label does not mean that the product contains no salt, but that there has not been any added to the original amount. Be especially cautious when buying canned goods, soy sauces, salted pretzels, nuts, crackers, olives, and pickles. A few extra minutes spent checking labels can be an eye opening experience.

I was shocked to find that one dill pickle can contain up to 1900 mg of sodium, but not so surprised to find that one MacDonald's Big Mac contains 950 mg of sodium. Most frozen dinners, pizza, and processed meats, such as bacon and hot dogs, contain extremely high levels of sodium. A single meal in a fast food restaurant can come close to meeting your sodium requirements for the whole day, which explains why many people feel bloated after eating fast foods.

The good news is that potassium naturally counter-balances sodium. Foods high in potassium are thought to positively affect the cardiovascular system by lowering blood pressure. When you increase your level of potassium rich foods, you naturally reduce the negative effects of excessive sodium.

The recommended daily intake for potassium is about 3,500 mg per day, which is far more than the typical American normally consumes. It is possible, however, to obtain too much potassium and excessive amounts may cause heart rhythm irregularities.

Since most fruits and vegetables contain significantly higher levels of potassium than sodium, you can naturally increase your potassium level simply by eating more of these Pura Vida lifestyle staples. Remember, fresher is usually better and steaming retains more nutrients than boiling. Some good sources of potassium include bananas, oranges, cantaloupe, papaya, watermelon, prunes, potatoes, lima beans, spinach, carrots, squash, tomatoes, and mushrooms.

We found that experimenting with and adding fresh herbs and various season-ings to our meals made it much easier to give up the saltshaker habit. It may take some time to discover which seasonings appeal to your particular taste buds, but once you do, you may be surprised to find that you completely lose your craving for salt.

The controversy over sodium and other nutrients will likely continue, and new data and research will continue to define what our society perceives as the truth. It can all be quite confusing and overwhelming. Some of the answers to your specific questions are apparent, however, if you simply become more informed and aware, and listen to your body's inner wisdom for guidance.

If your stomach hurts or you feel bloated after eating fast food, listen to that warning signal and learn from it. If your fingers or ankles swell or your eyes are puffy after eating high levels of salty foods, take that as an important message from your body.

These examples may seem obvious, but are warning signs that go unrecog-nized or ignored by millions of people who are in too much of a hurry to listen to their remarkably intelligent bodies. By taking the time to listen to your body and treat it with respect, you will find that the answers come much more easily and naturally, and that your sense of direction is much clearer and more focused.

Nutrition And Supplementation

As recently as a decade ago, the mysterious authority commonly called *they* claimed that taking vitamin and mineral supplements was a complete waste of time and money and only gave you expensive urine. During the majority of its history, conventional medicine has contested the importance of supplementing one's diet with vitamins and minerals, severely criticizing alternative practitioners who believed that nutritional factors were crucial in preventing and even curing disease.

It has only been in the past decade or so that conventional medical groups have jumped on the bandwagon, claiming as their own something that was once only in the domain of alternative practitioners from the United States and traditional practitioners in countries such as China, Japan, and India. Often these alternative nutritional beliefs and therapies have been passed down from generation to generation in Eastern medicine, some of them dating back thousands of years.

While, in the past, conventional medicine often violently opposed alternative therapies such as supplementation, a phenomenon has recently evolved that I like to think of as a changing tide in health care. Most medical practitioners now recognize the importance of nutrition in maintaining health and often work together with non-medical health providers in the best interests of their patients.

In my opinion, much more cooperation is needed, however, and until more funding is allocated for research and application of non-medical therapies, the public will continue to rely heavily on the medical community for the majority of its information and scientific data.

Some of the past controversy over supplementation stemmed partially from extravagant claims, such as those related to rapid weight loss or miraculous cancer cures, which are usually made by those with something to gain financially. As seen in so many other areas, the practical benefits of supplementation were often overshadowed by the sensationalism of a few opportunistic individuals.

There is still considerable debate in the scientific community about supplementation. As numerous research studies are continually proving, however, vitamins and minerals play a much bigger role in maintaining optimal health than was previously believed by conventional western medicine.

Today, it is widely accepted that certain nutrients can help prevent heart disease, birth defects, cataracts, and even cancer. We now know that a proper diet, including supplementation when needed, is essential to improving overall health and even slowing down the aging process.

What exactly do vitamins and minerals do? Vitamins play a role in converting food into energy and living tissues. They also help regulate the chemical reactions that protect the cells, and are essential for the release of energy in the body. Minerals are also necessary for the transformation of proteins, fats, and carbohydrates into energy. Minerals are an integral part of the process of building and maintaining the structure of the body.

Notice that the word energy is a key component of both of these definitions. Although vitamins and minerals are not a direct source of energy (as are proteins, carbohydrates, and fats) these substances are crucial components in metabolic processes resulting in energy.

Ideally, you should try to obtain the vitamins and minerals that your body needs through your daily diet, since food is the most efficient source of these nutrients. By eating a wide variety of high quality, fresh, whole foods, you increase your chances of obtaining all the vital health promoting nutrients.

Unfortunately, for a number of reasons, very few people manage to meet their optimal specific nutritional requirements through food alone. One reason is that the soil that our food is grown in is often depleted, due to the overuse of chemicals and fertilizers. Vitamins and minerals are also lost during the time it takes to transport food to the grocery stores, where your fruits and vegetables often sit for extended periods of time, causing them to lose even more nutrients.

Cooking also robs some food of valuable nutrients, although steaming generally retains more nutrients in your vegetables than boiling. The enzymes found in fresh fruits and vegetables are necessary for the proper digestion of food. These vital enzymes can be destroyed when they are heated, preventing the release of vitamins, minerals, and amino acids that are a crucial component in the energy producing process. Stress and smoking can also deplete the body of vital nutrients.

It is difficult to consume the exact combination and variety of foods necessary for optimal nutrition and peak energy. For these reasons I believe that supplementation is beneficial in providing your body with all the elements needed for optimal health.

However, it is a dangerous misconception that taking supplements is an adequate substitute for a poor diet. Taking vitamins does not make it acceptable to eat more processed, packaged food. Neither is it a good idea to use supplements in a prescription type manner while ignoring health related symptoms. As you know, there are no instant shortcuts to health, and pure health does not come in a bottle. The bottom line is there is no substitute for the nutrients found naturally in a balanced diet of a wide variety of fresh, wholesome foods.

Pay special attention to the food sources of vitamins and minerals, and keep them in mind the next time you do your grocery shopping. Remember, the daily decisions you make as you travel down your path are what transform information and knowledge into powerful actions. Something as routine as grocery shopping can change the direction that your life is headed in.

For example, when shopping for groceries, you should be aware that the term enriched does not always mean that a product is better for you than the original. When a product is enriched, something valuable was usually lost in the processing, and synthetically replaced or added.

For this reason, try to avoid products made with white or bleached flour. Whole wheat, rye, oat bran, or buckwheat flour are much healthier choices. When shopping, look specifically for bread that is labeled 100% whole wheat. Whole wheat bread has more than three times as much fiber, magnesium, chromium, vitamin E, and B6 than white bread. Pasta is a great source of complex carbohydrates; however, traditional white pasta lacks the vitamins and minerals found in whole wheat or spinach pasta.

The body produces a limited number of vitamins. For example, vitamin D is manufactured in the skin during exposure to sunlight. Certain vitamins and minerals work best when taken together. Vitamin C aids in the absorption of iron, and vitamin D helps calcium and phosphorous to be absorbed.

Vitamins are divided into two categories: fat soluble and water-soluble. Certain vitamins, such as A, D, E, and K, are considered fat-soluble. These vitamins are transported by the fats in the bloodstream, which is just one of the reasons why a healthy amount of dietary fat is needed for optimal nutrition.

Since vitamins A, D, E, and K are easily stored in body tissues, excessive intake of fat soluble vitamins can build up to toxic levels in your body. Water-soluble vitamins such as the B Complex vitamins, and vitamin C, are excreted in the urine and other body fluids. For this reason, they must be constantly provided through diet or supplementation.

Although it is possible to experience side effects from consuming too much of the water soluble vitamins, it is less likely to occur than over consumption of the fat soluble type. Do not assume that because something is good for you, more of it must be better for you. Please be aware that taking mega doses of vitamins, even the water-soluble type, is a common practice with potentially dangerous side effects. Vitamin B6, for example, can cause nerve damage when taken in excessive doses, and taking mega doses of ascorbic acid (vitamin C) over an extended period can contribute to kidney stones.

Supplements are best absorbed when taken with food. The higher quality the food is, the better the absorption. For this reason, it is most beneficial to take supplements after meals and space them out as evenly as possible throughout the day.

One of the wonderful things about humans is that, like snowflakes, no two people in the world are exactly alike. We are all biochemically unique individuals and have varying nutritional energy needs. For this reason, no two individuals have exactly the same daily vitamin and mineral requirements for optimal health.

The daily values (DV's) commonly used today, which were formerly known as RDAs, are simply overall guidelines for the general population. They do not necessarily represent the amounts needed for individual optimal health or the amounts needed to forestall chronic disease. These allowances are the amount of nutrients that, when acquired daily, are considered to be sufficient to meet the known nutritional needs of most healthy persons, and prevent severe deficiencies.

The strength of a certain vitamin is usually expressed in micrograms (ug) or milligrams (mg). Your specific requirements vary depending on your gender, age, activity level, overall physical condition, and body chemistry. Taking prescription or over the counter (OTC) drugs can also enter into the supplementation equation. These substances can deplete vital nutrients when taken on a regular basis. For example, aspirin can deplete the body's stores of vitamin C. Diuretics and some antibiotics can lower the levels of potassium in the body, and antacids containing aluminum can disturb delicate calcium and phosphorus levels.

Pay special attention to the vitamin and mineral content of the foods that you eat. You will find that certain foods, such as dark green leafy vegetables, seem to be a source of almost every healthy nutrient. Surprisingly, iceberg lettuce is mostly water and has little nutritional value compared to its dark green counterparts. You will also find that, in general, foods high in complex carbohydrates are also high in valuable nutrients.

Recently, there has been a great deal of excitement about a group of nutrients known as antioxidants that fight toxic molecules known as free radicals. Beta-carotene and the vitamins C and E, are powerful antioxidants. Free radicals are a natural byproduct of cell metabolism. They are also created in the body by exposure to tobacco smoke, sunlight, ozone, automobile exhaust, high fat diets, environmental pollutants, and lack of exercise.

When too many free radicals are circulating in the bloodstream, they can have harmful effects, roaming the cells, damaging DNA, corroding cell membranes, breaking down skin tissue, and even killing cells. These dangerous free radicals are thought to play a major role in the development of cancer, heart and lung disease, and even in accelerating the aging process. Fortunately, antioxidants are nature's way of neutralizing these harmful free radicals.

By making an effort to consume specific types of foods, you may be protecting yourself from the devastating effects of cancer. It is believed that some colorful foods such as carrots, broccoli, and green leafy vegetables (all rich in vitamin A) have anti-cancer properties.

Certain vegetables, such as brussel sprouts and cauliflower, are thought to have similar benefits as well. In the following chapter, I will discuss specific dietary sources of the anti-cancer ACES: A (beta carotene), C, E, and Selenium.

As you can see, the issue of supplementation is an exciting but somewhat complicated matter that should not be taken lightly. For this reason, I urge you to do ongoing research on your own in addition to reading this book, in order to fully educate yourself about the ever-changing area of supplementation. It is quite possible that you will find the answer to some specific health problems you are experiencing by researching the benefits of a certain vitamin or mineral.

For even more specific nutritional advice, talk to the health care provider of your choice. It will take some time to get the complete picture about your specific requirements and needs. The time and energy you spend working toward this goal, however, will be well worth the return investment.

Len and I have been taking supplements since we were young adults and believe that supplementing our healthy diets with vitamins and minerals is an excellent way to fill in the nutritional gaps and increase our chances of living longer, healthier, more energetic lives. Speaking from experience, we can honestly say that we believe that taking supplements throughout our lives has improved the quality of our journey and helped us live our lives at our full potential.

Personally, I have always taken a high quality vitamin and multi mineral supplement, yet the individual, additional supplements that I have taken along with it have varied throughout the years. Part of the reason for this is that I often add or subtract a certain nutrient for a few months to see if I notice a difference in my body with or without that specific nutrient. My specific intake has also changed as I age and as my level of nutritional awareness evolves.

You can usually find high quality supplements at your local health food store, which I prefer over drug or retail store brands. I often order our supplements, protein powders, and sports bars from catalogues and have found that they are generally less expensive when purchased in higher quantities.

One of my favorite energy boosters comes in the form of highly concentrated, nutrient-rich food powders sometimes known as green drinks or natural greens. The power packed fruit and vegetable based powders can be mixed with water or your favorite juice for a natural supplement to your diet and are a potent source of vitamins, minerals, enzymes, antioxidants, fiber and the essential amino acids.

The ones that I like best contain ingredients such as barley grass, wheat grass, spirulina, and non-dairy probiotics that can strengthen the immune system and neutralize toxins. The impressive list of ingredients and phytochemicals originally got my attention but the proof is in the way these greens make you feel.

I believe that powdered greens are partially responsible for my productive morning energy and increased mental alertness. I went for a few days without them recently and noticed a big dip in my energy level and stamina at the gym. They taste much better than they look and are perfect for grabbing on your way out the door and drinking in the car. Simply spoon them into a large mouthed water bottle with some water or juice and shake vigorously.

If you have never taken vitamins or minerals, or only taken supplements sporadically, you may simply want to start out by consistently taking a high quality multi-vitamin/mineral supplement. Over time, you can gradually add specific nutrients, such as antioxidants or herbal supplements.

As with every other aspect of your constantly evolving Pura Vida lifestyle, it is important to listen to your body's innate intelligence when supplementing your diet. Pay close attention to messages from your digestive system, energy level, and immune system while adding to or making changes in your vitamin and mineral consumption.

For all of the reasons listed in this chapter and more, the practice of taking supplements wisely is the next helpful stepping stone on your Pura Vida path.

Stepping Stone #11: *Pay special attention to the feedback that your body gives you as you supplement your healthy diet with high quality vitamins and minerals.*

When fully integrated with all the other helpful stepping stones along your path thus far, supplementation can be the added impetus you may need to help you overcome life's hurdles in what sometimes seems like a challenging obstacle course. I hope that the following nutritional information that I have gathered along my own personal path will aid you in your own quest for the truth and help you to lead a fuller, more energetic life.

Vitamins

To help you become more familiar with some of the most important vitamins and minerals, I have provided the following basic information. Keep in mind that this is only a partial list and that every day new discoveries are being made. I suggest using the next two chapters as a quick reference guide. Instead of trying to memorize the information, you may want to lightly read it over and refer back later as needed, so that you do not lose your steady momentum.

VITAMIN OVERVIEW

I find beta-carotene, which is also called pro-vitamin A, particularly interesting because beta carotene is turned into vitamin A by the body as needed. Although vitamin A can cause toxicity in mega doses, beta carotene does not, since the body will not convert beta carotene into Vitamin A unless it has a specific need for it.

Beta-carotene is found naturally in orange fruits and vegetables, such as carrots, sweet potatoes, and cantaloupes, and in dark green, leafy vegetables, such as spinach and collard greens. In recent years, beta-carotene has attracted worldwide attention from scientists, who are investigating its positive effects on heart disease, cataracts, cancer, and the various aspects of aging.

Vitamin A, also known as retinol, is a fat-soluble vitamin that positively affects the function of the immune system and improves eyesight, especially night vision. Many of the traditional sources of vitamin A, such as liver, beef, and eggs, are high in cholesterol and fat. Fortunately, however, you can increase your intake of vitamin A by consuming more of the beta carotene-rich fruit and vegetable sources listed above. Your marvelous, innately intelligent body will convert beta-carotene to vitamin A as it is needed.

Vitamin B-1, B-2, B-3, B-6, B-12, and folic acid are among the vital B complex vitamins. I like to think of the B complex vitamins as the Pure Energy Vitamins because they play a crucial role in helping to release energy from food, and are extremely important in the metabolism of proteins, carbohydrates, and fats.

B vitamins are involved in nearly every reaction in the body, and some of the B complex vitamins may also help fight cancer and strengthen the immune system. The B vitamins are water soluble and can also be depleted by stress. They should be taken together for optimal benefits.

Vitamin B-1, or thiamine, is a necessary component in the production of energy. Alcoholics are especially prone to vitamin B-1 deficiency since alcohol impedes the body's ability to process thiamine. Some good sources of thiamine are whole grains such as oatmeal, rice, and whole wheat, legumes, nuts, eggs, milk, fish, wheat germ, salmon, navy and kidney beans.

Vitamin B-2, also known as riboflavin, is involved in helping the body burn fats, carbohydrates, and proteins, and is necessary for maintaining healthy mucous membranes. A riboflavin deficiency can show up as cracks at the corners of the mouth and itching and burning of the eyes. Skim milk is an excellent source of riboflavin. Eggs, lean meats, poultry, whole grain breads and cereals, dairy products, and yeast are all good sources of vitamin B-2.

Vitamin B-3 or niacin is also important in the metabolic process. Niacin increases circulation and helps keep the digestive system healthy. It is sometimes used to help prevent premenstrual headaches, and to treat dizziness and ringing in the ears.

Sometimes, taking too much niacin or taking it on an empty stomach can produce a reaction commonly known as niacin flush, which causes your skin to turn bright red and can be quite uncomfortable.

I have personally experienced this unpleasant side effect when I was younger and took Niacin on a nearly empty stomach. My skin turned so red that my friend's mother wanted to take me to the emergency room. It seemed funny afterward but was quite alarming at the time.

A certain form of Vitamin B-3, known as nicotinic acid (not to be confused with nicotine) may lower the amount of cholesterol and triglycerides in the blood, reducing the risk of heart disease. Some natural sources of niacin are the lean white meat of chicken and turkey, fish, legumes, and whole grains.

Vitamin B-6 or pyroxidine has a multitude of functions, including helping the body process proteins, carbohydrates, and fats. Pyroxidine also works with other vitamins and minerals to supply the energy used in muscles.

Pyroxidine aids in the production of red blood cells and the cells of the immune system. Vitamin B-6 affects almost every system of the body, and may help relieve the symptoms of PMS, morning sickness, and carpal tunnel syndrome.

Vitamin B-6 also helps the body resist stress. Fish, brown rice, cereal grains, brewer's yeast, wheat germ, the white meat of chicken, bananas, broccoli, salmon, and tuna, are just some of the natural sources of B-6.

Vitamin B-12, also known as cobalamine or cyanocobalamine, is essential in the formation and regeneration of red blood cells and helps prevent anemia. B-12 is only obtained from animal sources such as poultry, eggs, fish, and milk.

Vegans (people who do not eat food that comes from animals) should supplement their diet with B-12, since it cannot be obtained from plant-based foods. Some good sources for B-12 are low fat dairy products, chicken, turkey, shrimp and salmon.

Another extremely promising B complex vitamin, folic acid, works hand in hand with B-12. Folic acid is necessary for the formation of red blood cells, and has been linked to the prevention of certain types of birth defects. Dark green leafy vegetables such as spinach, and wheat germ, citrus fruits and beans are excellent sources of folic acid.

Pregnant women and women planning to conceive should make an effort to obtain sufficient amounts of folic acid, since it is crucial to have adequate amounts of folic acid in the mother's body during the first few weeks of pregnancy. Folic acid helps regulate nerve cell development in the embryo and also in the developing baby. Folic acid's role in preventing serious birth defects is so crucial that the FDA will soon require that it be added to some foods.

Possibly my favorite vitamin, Vitamin C, is a potent antioxidant with a multitude of health promoting properties. The chemical name for vitamin C is ascorbic acid. This powerful vitamin has been linked with everything from the prevention of lung, breast, colon, and cervical cancer and the reduction of cholesterol, to reducing the risk of cataracts and preventing colds. In addition, Vitamin C is essential in wound healing and the formation of collagen. It has been linked to the prevention of skin cancers and wrinkles that result from exposure to ultraviolet rays, as well.

It is very important to maintain a high level of vitamin C in the bloodstream, since stress, smoking, and environmental pollutants can destroy it. Women who take oral contraceptives also have an increased need for this vital nutrient.

Since vitamin C is water soluble and quickly excreted through the urine, it is necessary to replenish your stores by frequently eating fresh fruits and vegetables, and taking supplements if needed. I often recommend taking timed-release vitamin C or splitting the dosage by taking morning and evening supplements.

Vitamin C has been proven to boost immunity and studies have indicated that it can help prevent and decrease the symptoms of the common cold. I have personally experienced the powerful effects of large doses of vitamin C on the immune system but do not recommend taking mega doses over an extended period of time. Even though ascorbic acid is water soluble, excessive intake can cause kidney stones and gastrointestinal disturbances such as diarrhea.

Citrus fruits such as oranges and grapefruits, and dark green vegetables, tomatoes, potatoes, broccoli, strawberries, cantaloupe, and green peppers are all excellent sources of vitamin C.

Vitamin D is nicknamed the sunshine vitamin because your body can manufacture vitamin D after being exposed to the sun. It is necessary for the proper formation of teeth and bones, and is a vital component in proper functioning of the nervous system. Vitamin D also helps maintain the correct ratio of calcium and phosphorus in the blood.

In order for calcium to be properly absorbed from food, vitamin D must be present. Like other fat soluble vitamins, Vitamin D can be toxic in long term mega doses. Some natural sources of Vitamin D are sunshine, skim milk, dairy products, salmon, sardines, and wheat germ.

Vitamin E, also known as alpha tocopherol, is thought to slow down the aging process by preventing oxidative damage to the cells. Alpha tocopherol has been linked to reduced plaque buildup in coronary arteries, thus lowering the risk of heart disease.

Vitamin E has also been linked to the prevention of breast, colon, lung and prostate cancer. I have found through practical experience that this amazing fat-soluble vitamin works wonders on the skin, speeding up the healing process of burns and decreasing scar tissue. I recommend keeping a bottle of Vitamin E oil, which can be purchased at most health food stores and some drug stores, in your medicine cabinet for use on damaged skin.

Vitamin E is found naturally in vegetable oils, whole grains, nuts, seeds, green leafy vegetables, legumes, and wheat germ. You should be aware that mega doses in excessive amounts can actually alter the immune system and impair sexual function.

Vitamin K, another fat-soluble vitamin, is interesting in that one form of this vitamin is produced in the body by friendly bacteria that are found in the intestinal tract. Vitamin K is a necessary element in blood clotting and helps prevent abnormal bleeding, and is found naturally in spinach, cauliflower, oats, cabbage, green tea, and soybeans.

Minerals From The Earth

Since we are all integrally connected to our environment, it seems only fitting that many of the minerals naturally found on the earth's crust are necessary for the formation of our body's structure and for the miraculous transformation of food into energy.

Vitamins and minerals work hand in hand and most vitamins cannot work without the aid of minerals. Certain minerals, known as electrolytes, maintain the proper delicate balance of fluids in the body.

One of the most important and abundant minerals in your body is calcium, 99 perent of which is found in your bones and teeth. The other 1 percent is found in body fluids and tissues. Not only does calcium help build and maintain bones and teeth, but calcium also must be present in precisely the right amount to help nerves send messages, to regulate cellular fluids, and to help the blood clot and the heart beat.

Interestingly, although calcium is the most abundant mineral in the body, calcium deficiency is the most common of the mineral deficiencies. Osteoporosis, the sometimes crippling bone disease that affects approximately one in four post-menopausal women, is characterized by a loss of calcium and phosphorus from the inner part of the bones.

Although the exact cause of osteoporosis is not known, dietary deficiencies and hormonal changes are thought to be contributing factors. This condition, which can also affect men, causes the bones to lose their density and makes them thin, fragile, and more susceptible to fractures. The good news is that by consuming the proper amounts of calcium throughout your life, you can help minimize the risk of bone loss associated with osteoporosis.

Some other positive news is that exercise stimulates bone growth, and can help prevent osteoporosis by increasing bone mass. Weight bearing exercises such as walking and weight training appear to be more effective in preventing osteoporosis than non-weight bearing exercises such as swimming.

Both high fiber foods and iron supplements can inhibit your body's absorption of calcium. For this reason, you should not take calcium and iron together or take calcium supplements after eating a particularly high fiber food such as bran cereal. Also, keep in mind that vitamin D is necessary for the absorption of calcium.

Since some of the long-term effects of osteoporosis are irreversible, prevention is truly the key. Keep in mind that smoking, caffeine, sugar, and alcohol can deplete your body's stores of calcium. One way to avoid calcium loss may be to cut back on excessive consumption of sodas containing phosphoric acid.

Calcium is found naturally in green leafy vegetables such as kale and turnip greens, which actually are quite tasty when steamed. It is also found in salmon and sardines, molasses, broccoli, snow peas, soybeans, and figs. Perhaps the best known source of calcium is dairy products, including skim milk, yogurt, and cottage cheese.

Women in particular sometimes avoid dairy products in an effort to cut back on calories. Often, they will choose diet soft drinks over calcium rich skim milk without realizing the detrimental effects the choice may eventually have on their bones and their bodies.

Luckily, due to the current availability of most dairy products in low fat and fat free versions, your bones can benefit from these calcium rich choices without adding inches to your hips, thighs, and stomach.

I have always liked the passage in the bible that states, "A merry heart doeth good like a medicine, but a broken spirit drieth the bones." I can personally vouch for the merry heart doing good part, and also believe there may be a connection between depression and similar negative emotions and the debilitating condition of osteoporosis. As a result of my clinical experience, I also have noticed that people who are depressed are less active and less likely to engage in weight bearing activities such as walking, running, and weight lifting, which stimulate bone growth.

If you are having trouble giving up junk food or soft drinks, or starting a regular exercise program, talking to a woman who has a dowager's hump on her curved back or meeting someone who has suffered through the ordeal of a fractured pelvis, could be the impetus that makes you want to create these positive changes in your life.

Iron is another vital mineral that is very often deficient in the diet. This mineral is necessary to create the protein hemoglobin, which carries oxygen-rich blood from the lungs to all the tissues of the body. Iron is also important in the conversion of food to energy.

Since the mineral iron is involved in both the transportation of oxygen and the creation of energy, it is easy to see why one of the main signs of iron deficiency is fatigue. Insufficient amounts of iron also adversely affect the immune system, brain function, and physical endurance. Menstruation, pregnancy, and breast-feeding can all increase the body's demand for iron.

Vegans and vegetarians should be careful to obtain sufficient amounts of this vital mineral, and should also be aware that iron from plant sources, such as green leafy vegetables, is not well absorbed by the body. The body absorbs *heme* iron that comes from animal sources, more efficiently.

The food source for the most absorbable iron is meat; however, to obtain the proper amounts of iron, it is not necessary to eat large quantities of saturated fat filled red meat. Some of my favorite dietary sources of iron include the white meat of chicken or turkey, wheat germ, nuts, molasses, egg whites, whole grains, raisins, prune juice, and dried beans.

Another crucial mineral, magnesium, is thought to have a protective effect on the heart, and is sometimes used in hospitals to treat heart rhythm abnormalities. Calcium and magnesium should be taken together because magnesium regulates calcium uptake by the cells. Some good sources of magnesium are those green leafy vegetables once again, seafood, garbanzo beans, almonds, bananas, whole grains, and wheat bran.

As I explained earlier, the mineral potassium is essential in the balancing of cellular fluids. It also plays a vital role in maintaining proper heart rhythm. Like many other minerals, potassium helps release energy from proteins, carbohydrates, and fats. Both potassium and sodium are important in the elimination of cellular wastes.

Although bananas are the most well known source of potassium, green leafy vegetables, potatoes, citrus fruits, whole grain cereals, carrots, lima beans, and squash are also all good sources of potassium.

Selenium is an interesting antioxidant that is thought to strengthen the immune system and boost the antioxidant activities of vitamin E. Selenium helps slow the aging process by preventing tissue damage due to oxidation. Selenium also helps retain the elasticity of skin and other body tissue.

A severe deficiency of selenium can lead to premature aging and male infertility. Selenium-rich foods include whole grains and bran, tomatoes, onions, broccoli, seafood, garlic, chicken, and tuna. Please be aware that long term excessive supplementation of selenium can result in toxicity.

Even though zinc is a trace mineral, it is still necessary for most functions in the body, including bone formation, wound healing, immunity, and the production of energy. Zinc also helps preserve our senses of taste and smell. Zinc deficiencies are often found in patients with diabetes, prostate, and throat cancers. Negative effects on the immune system, such as decreased antibody response and reduction of the number and function of infection fighting lymphocytes, can be a result of inadequate levels of zinc.

Zinc is best known for its reputation for helping to prevent the common cold. Although eating foods rich in zinc should give your immune system a boost, you should be aware that taking mega doses of zinc supplements can actually decrease immunity.

Similar to the mineral iron, zinc found in animal protein is absorbed more efficiently than that which comes from plant sources. Oysters and crab meat are particularly high in zinc. The lean white meat of chicken or turkey, wheat germ, whole grains, legumes, nuts, seeds, and blackstrap molasses are good sources of zinc.

Recently, the trace mineral chromium has been very popular with the health club crowd and those wanting to lose weight. Chromium is one of the main ingredients in many of the new natural products claiming to help you lose body-fat and increase muscle. It is estimated that 90 percent of Americans are deficient in this nutrient.

Chromium makes it easier for the body to burn glucose. Insulin (which is vital for regulating the metabolism of carbohydrates, proteins, and fats) works better in the presence of chromium. Insulin also affects our bodies by regulating blood sugar levels and cannot perform its job properly without chromium. Diets high in simple sugars deplete chromium from the body. Chromium may also improve the symptoms of the type of diabetes that develops in older adults.

Chromium picolinate is a supplemental form of chromium that is easily used by the body. It has been linked to the reduction of elevated cholesterol, and in some limited studies it has been linked to the reduction of body fat accompanied by an increase in lean muscle mass.

Most of the fantastic fat burning claims concerning this mineral sound too good to be true, and probably are. The research is still fairly new and much more is needed. As you already know, there is no magic pill that eliminates bodyfat and dramatically increases muscle.

Another one of the common ingredients in natural weight loss products is the amino acid carnitine. Many athletes have been supplementing their diet with carnitine for years because they feel that it is a performance enhancer that facilitates longer, more strenuous workouts. Scientific research validating this claim, however, is also limited.

It is known that carnitine is essential in helping the body to burn fat because it transfers fatty acids into cells where they are converted into energy. Energy from fats, carbohydrates, and proteins is released from inside cells by the powerhouse of the cell, which is called the mitochondria. To enter the powerhouse, fats must be transported by the carnitine shuttle. Fats can only be converted into energy if carnitine is present.

It remains to be seen if these supplements and the similar products that will inevitably follow are the revolutionary fat burning breakthroughs that some manufacturers would like you to believe. In my opinion, the advertisements for these so-called fat burning products are often misleading and give consumers false hope.

In fact, many widely advertised and extremely popular weight loss products can actually be harmful, especially if they contain the ingredient known as ephedra. Also known as ma huang, ephedra raises blood pressure and puts stress on the circulatory system. The potential for health related risks is so high that as of April, 2004, the FDA officially banned buying or selling a dietary supplement containing ephedra.

On the other end of the spectrum is a popular supplement that I personally feel shows great promise in the area of easing the symptoms of osteoarthritis and perhaps even slowing its progression. Glucosamine is a natural substance produced by the body and found primarily in joint cartilage, where it is thought to maintain an important role in maintaining joint health and resilience. Glucosamine and chondroitin have developed a large following among arthritis sufferers and are frequently recommended by almost every holistic nutritional expert and orthopedic surgeon that I personally know as a first line of defense in maintaining joint health.

Although these nutrients do play a vital role in optimal health, they are only one piece of the puzzle. There is no substitute for proper nutrition, eating fresh whole foods, regular exercise, and all the other pieces that make the Pura Vida picture complete.

Mother Nature's Secrets

Throughout history, most cultures have used gifts from Mother Nature, including herbs, plants, and foods, for their health promoting, curative, and preventive properties with great success. Sometimes referred to as secret family remedies, these natural gifts have frequently been passed down through many generations and are often quite effective.

One excellent example of a natural remedy that has been proven to be nutritionally beneficial is the odiferous bulb, garlic, which improves the function of the immune system and is also thought to have antioxidant effects.

Research suggests that garlic may improve cardiovascular health and offer protective effects against cancer. Raw garlic and its relatives (onions, leeks, chives, and scallions) contain allyl sulfides, which may help rid the body of carcinogens and depress the growth of cancer cells.

Garlic has also been shown to lower total cholesterol and raise HDL levels, prevent blood clots from forming, and lower blood pressure. Because of its blood thinning properties, people who regularly take anticoagulant drugs or aspirin should consult their doctor before adding large amounts of garlic to their diet.

Garlic is just one of an exciting list of foods containing phytochemicals (a group of chemicals found in plants) presently being studied by the National Cancer Institute for their health promoting properties. The special chemicals found in garlic, citrus fruits, celery, soybeans, ginger root, hot peppers, green tea, and licorice root may help prevent cancer and other diseases.

Another interesting group of vegetables, named cruciferous, contains high levels of phytochemicals and is thought to discourage the development of cancer. Broccoli, cauliflower, kale, bok choy, swiss chard, and brussel sprouts are included in this classification of plants.

Due largely to increased public awareness of holistic and alternative health care, natural herbs have gained an astounding level of popularity in recent years. It is important to remember that these powerful gifts from the earth should be used with caution and treated with respect, however.

Although it seems that claims related to herbs are sometimes exaggerated, we personally have experienced some interesting positive results from nature's herbal remedies throughout our lives. Our interest was heightened while in the rainforest, which is the source of a very large percentage of the world's medicine.

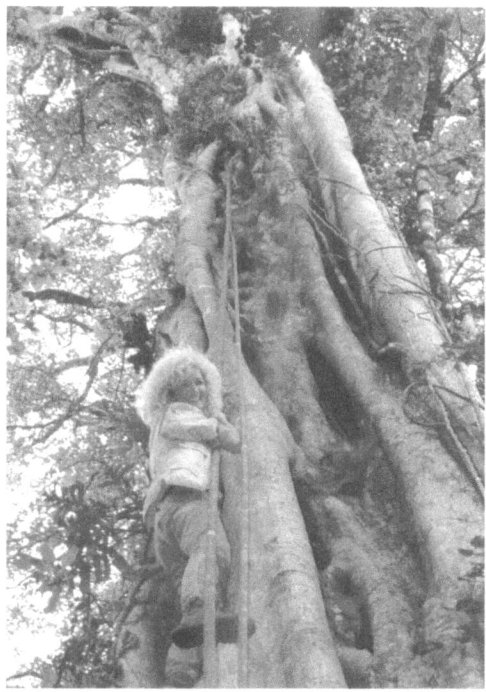

We had an interesting experience in Costa Rica after Len developed a painful ear infection while swimming in the pools of a waterfall deep in the jungle. We told a wise, motherly Tico friend of ours about Len's condition. We affectionately called this hearty, fun loving character Cookie because she was the baker of the home made oatmeal cookies from the synchronous sign earlier in our journey.

As soon as we told her, Cookie took us by the arm and led us through thick green foliage to her fragrant herb garden tucked away at the edge of the rainforest. There, she plucked a few leaves, crushed them, wrapped them in gauze, and instructed Len to place the concoction in his ear. The results were impressive. Within minutes, there was a significant decrease in the pain in his ear and the infection cleared up after repeated use within a few days.

This experience piqued our natural curiosity. During the remainder of our stay at Cookie's lodge, Villa Verde, on the outskirts of the Monteverde Biological

Reserve, we continued to follow her through the morning mist, asking questions as she pointed out fascinating plants and herbs which are commonly used to treat everything from migraine headaches to digestive disturbances.

Perhaps this experience was what opened us to the possibility of visiting a Chinese Doctor, which we did at the urging of another truly wise, spiritual friend while traveling in Chicago. The wizened, gentle healer with a flowing, long white beard was considered by some to be the unofficial Emperor of Chinatown in this windy city. He certainly looked the part as he sat in his simple store/office surrounded by many members of his family, including his beautiful, bright-eyed grandchildren.

With his daughter attempting translation, he asked us to stick out our tongues, and in demonstrating, stuck his own tongue out. We were both impressed by how pink and healthy looking this ancient man's tongue was. He also felt our pulses for quite some time and looked into our eyes.

Within a few short minutes, he was able to pinpoint the exact location of our problem areas, minor aches and pains, and recommended that we make teas from certain herbs in wooden bins packaged by shy, smiling members of his family in the outer area of his office. Our individual packages were a visually fascinating potpourri of barks, roots, berries, and other unidentifiable ingredients.

We tried, to no avail, to find out the names of the mysterious ingredients, but time was limited and the language barrier was too great. Instead of using our usual cautious, analytical approach, we chose to trust in the ancient wisdom of this highly respected little man, whose knowledge had been passed down through the centuries from chosen members of his ancestors.

Upon returning home, we boiled the teas as we had been instructed, and held our noses while drinking the nasty tasting liquid. We both can honestly say that there was a considerable difference in our energy levels during the time that we were drinking the stinky teas. The result was not the frenetic energy buzz that caffeine provides before taking a nosedive, but rather a balanced, calm, clear, and steady feeling.

As a result of these experiences and other similar adventures, I have continued to explore the healing power of herbs and research the exciting scientific information available concerning vitamins, minerals, and supplementation. I do not, however, consider myself to be an expert in these areas, only a seeker of my own personal truth, which I enjoy sharing with others.

In all honesty, it is sometimes hard for me to digest and remember all of the numbers and facts, but I continue to record them because I know that they will be meaningful to certain people on a similar path.

Whether you decide to continue your own ongoing research in this area or consult a traditional or alternative health care provider, it is important that you take the majority of the responsibility for your nutritional decisions and the state of your own health.

Rather than allowing yourself to become overwhelmed by the sheer volume of information available today, take time to listen to your inner being, as it shifts and reforms, continually growing and expanding. Slowly integrate the new information and ideas into your lifestyle and you will find new connections, surprising linkages that direct you on to new pathways.

I thoroughly enjoy all the benefits of living in our modern technological society. However, it seems we could all learn valuable lessons from the secrets of the natural world that have been passed down through the generations by people who protect and truly respect the earth.

Our experiences in the rainforest also reminded me that when we harm the earth, we are harming ourselves. Just as our minds, bodies, and spirits are profoundly interconnected, the human race is deeply connected to and dependent on our fragile earth. As bulldozers and fires continue to destroy the Amazon and other ancient rainforests at an alarmingly rapid rate, ripping immense patches out of their smooth green blankets of trees, we are all witnessing the permanent destruction of some of the largest, most mysterious and biologically diverse wilderness areas on Earth.

Sadly, only a small fraction of these mystical areas have been analyzed for pharmacological potential. As a result, many of Mother Nature's secrets are lost to us forever, perhaps even natural cures for cancer and other devastating, incurable diseases.

We can only hope that as more individuals and groups increase their levels of awareness and become more closely connected to the earth, there will be an increased effort to save what is left of our world's valuable, irreplaceable wilderness areas and the health and pure life promoting gifts contained within them.

Women And Excess Bodyfat

NOTE: This section was written specifically for women who want to learn more about reducing the lumps and bulges that are commonly referred to as cellulite. I hope this information answers some of your questions. If this subject is not of interest to you, please feel free to move on to the next chapter.

There has been considerable debate through the years over exactly what cellulite is. For all practical purposes, what is commonly called cellulite is simply excess adipose tissue or bodyfat, not some unique type of tissue.

Due to natural physiological differences, women normally have more bodyfat than men and the excess is stored in different areas, namely the hips, thighs, and buttocks. The distribution of a woman's fat deposits is determined largely by hormones, which play a major role in the buildup of excess bodyfat.

As a natural consequence of an imbalance in the pure energy equation, when you take in more food than your body needs to function, what is not needed for energy is stored as bodyfat. Over time, this excess can take on a lumpy, bulging appearance. It is at this stage that women commonly refer to the dimpled tissue as cellulite.

The main reason that fatty tissue has a different appearance in women than men is that women have thinner skin. A widely accepted theory is that the dimply appearance is due to fat pushing up between restrictions formed by connective tissue that separates the fat cells into small compartments, giving the visible fat a lumpy appearance under the skin.

In addition, as a woman ages, the skin begins to lose its elasticity and the underlying supporting network of fibers gradually loses its resiliency. Regardless of what name excess body fat goes by, it is basically another indicator or warning sign letting you know that something is out of balance in your lifestyle.

Although cottage cheese thighs and bellies may seem like an unimportant, cosmetic concern to some, having an abnormal amount of excess bodyfat represents a very real, unhealthy, confidence-eroding problem for millions of women. For many women, having a large amount of excess body fat is a constant source of frustration that can make trying on a swimsuit a traumatic, depressing experience. Excessive bodyfat can also have such a negative effect on a woman's self-confidence that she is embarrassed to participate in activities that would help reduce the problem.

As a woman who has experienced fluctuations in body fat levels throughout her life, I can personally sympathize with anyone who feels that fighting cellulite is a never-ending battle. What is commonly called cellulite is a very frequent topic of conversation among women and a source of enormous profit for a few opportunists promising miracle cures. When it comes to this situation, however, there are no miracle cures.

The simple truth is that there is no single, isolated factor that is solely responsible for causing excess bodyfat to accumulate. It is necessary to evaluate each aspect of your lifestyle individually, and make positive, permanent changes, when needed, in your overall lifestyle—not just one part of it.

It is very important to remember that having some bodyfat is healthy and physiologically necessary. This important component of our body's structure gives the female form its sensual, attractive curves and softness. As I often have to remind myself, you are not unfit or unhealthy simply because you have some visible fat or jiggly areas.

Be cautious of crossing over the line toward unhealthy obsession when it comes to losing bodyfat. Keep in mind that the half starved waifs smiling seductively from the pages of the fashion magazines often sacrifice their health and sometimes risk their lives to maintain their physical appearance.

Also keep in mind that the images we see in magazines and advertisements have been digitally altered so much that they sometimes bear little resemblance to the real thing. Try not to lose sight of the fact that true, optimal health comes from the inside.

So what if you do not have a perfect, rock hard body? You can start feeling good about your true self right now, knowing that you are treating your body with the respect it deserves. When you lovingly nourish your body and soul and strive to maintain a healthy balance in your life, people will notice it in your attitude, your eyes, and even your smile.

In today's world, it can be hard to find time to squeeze in the things that you instinctively know are good for you. You may be thinking "But it's just so hard. I barely have enough time and energy to clean the house, go grocery shopping, cook dinner, do laundry, and take care of everything else as it is." It is truly amazing that women get so much done in twenty-four hours, and wake up the next day and do it all again.

Caught up in the swirl of your superwoman days, it is easy to forget this simple truth; by doing all the things you need to do to eliminate excess body fat, you will create more energy to get through those long days, and make your journey through life more enjoyable along the way.

There will always be hurdles and stumbling blocks along your path to health. There may be times when you feel that rather than living your life, you are simply struggling to survive. At times like these, the quality of your health often becomes a low priority.

Another time when taking care of yourself often takes a back burner is during the low points of the female menstrual cycle. Unfortunately, the negative effects of ignoring your health during these challenging times are cumulative and can become part of a vicious cycle. You may be familiar with the cycle. You overeat or eat poorly because you are feeling a little down, which causes you to gain weight, which makes you even more depressed, which causes you to eat more.

The good news is that exercise can help curb your appetite and break this negative cycle. Consistent exercise can result in a marked improvement in your emotional health and even decrease premenstrual symptoms. You will find yourself with more energy to deal with the kids or the bills, and discover an increased sense of self-confidence and inner strength when exercise, movement and physical activity are an integral part of your everyday lifestyle.

Unfortunately, the food cravings that sometimes sabotage an otherwise healthy diet are an inevitable part of being a woman. Keep in mind, however, that most food cravings usually begin to fade after four to twelve minutes. When you experience an unhealthy food craving, it helps to divert your attention immediately to something else. Drink a glass of water, eat something healthy, talk to a friend, putter around the house, go for a walk, or pamper yourself.

Have a mental conversation with yourself and explain that if you eat one or two of those little chocolate chip cookies (which can easily turn into five or six) you will be consuming X grams of fat and empty calories. You will also be taking in simple sugars, chemicals, and preservatives, which negatively affect your body chemistry and can intensify mood swings. Remind yourself that you will probably feel guilty and disappointed with yourself soon after, indirectly affecting all other aspects of your life. Think of those cookies going straight to your hips, adding another dimple or bulge.

If you have noticed a positive difference in your energy level or in the way your clothes fit since making healthy changes in your lifestyle, tell your friends about it. Being a positive example for others reinforces your own goals, and gives you a clearer, more focused direction as you move forward on your unique path through life.

Another unique challenge facing women is the accumulation of excess bodyfat that often accompanies pregnancy. Due to hormonal changes, it is perfectly normal and healthy to gain weight during pregnancy. Unfortunately, by trying to ensure that the baby will be well nourished, many women often overeat, or eat too much of the wrong kinds of foods. A variety of wholesome, nutritious foods with high vitamin, mineral and fiber content are what is important during this special time. Think quality and content.

Also, do not accept the mindset that because many of the women in your family have excess body fat, you are destined to carry excessive weight around for the rest of your life as well. Although heredity does play some part, it is possible that you have inherited some of their bad habits and lifestyle choices along with their genes.

Now we come to the question that often comes up when the word cellulite is mentioned. "What about the cellulite creams available on the market today?" Wouldn't it be wonderful if there were some miracle product that we could rub on our problem areas for a few minutes that made them all vanish? Of course, nothing in life is ever that simple.

When you read the fine print of most anti-cellulite products, you will find phrases such as "This product should be used in conjunction with an exercise program and proper nutrition." Supposedly, by improving the condition of the skin and underlying supportive tissue, most manufacturers only claim to reduce the *appearance* of cellulite, not the cellulite itself.

In my opinion, the time, money, and energy invested in using cellulite creams and similar products could be better spent on understanding what specifically causes you to accumulate excess body fat. Use that time to begin taking a positive, lasting course of action toward improving the way you feel about your problem areas.

If inactivity or excessive sitting has caused your backside to flatten or widen, it is important to concentrate on reshaping and rebuilding the musculature in the areas where muscle tissue has become flabby or jiggly.

Increasingly, today's lifestyles involve too much sitting. Your body was not made to sit as often as many of us do, whether it is in our cars, at work, at home on the couch and in the kitchen, or in restaurants. An inactive lifestyle which involves a great deal of sitting eventually causes the gluteal (buttocks) muscles to lose their tone and encourages more fat to accumulate in women's hips and thighs. The more you have to sit, the more active you should try to be when you have a choice not to sit.

Also, knowing the location and function of your lower body muscles helps you to isolate specific muscle groups in your problem areas. The exercises I have recommended are ones that I have found to be the most effective for strengthening and reshaping weak, flabby muscles, and rebuilding the structure underneath the fat deposits, making them appear smoother and less noticeable.

The excess bodyfat that is stored around the hips, thighs, and buttocks, is actually subcutaneous fat. The location of these deposits of fat is between the skin and the muscles. Although there is such a thing as intramuscular fat (similar to what gives red meat its marbled appearance), most of a woman's excess body fat is stored in this subcutaneous layer. That is why it is possible to have large muscles hiding under a layer of fat that are simply waiting to pop out and be seen as soon as you reduce excess bodyfat.

Subcutaneous fat is distinctly separate from the muscle groups. You cannot specifically reduce your stores of fat from a single area such as the hips or thighs by exercising only those areas because your body burns fat from the whole system. If the body's fuel needs are great enough, however, you will eventually lose in the desired area.

Something that I found very interesting in my research is that, in general, there is an order to the process of accumulation of bodyfat in women. Excess body fat usually starts to build up first on the back of the thigh and then the outer part of the thigh. Next it will accumulate in the hip region, before progressing to the stage involving the stomach and upper body, particularly the triceps, in the back of the upper arm.

Most of the time, women lose bodyfat in the reverse order; upper body first, then eventually down to the backs of the thighs. The hormone estrogen helps deposit fat in the hips, thighs, and buttocks, and fat in these areas is metabolized more slowly than in other areas.

Unfair as it may seem, it is easier for a man to lose excess weight in his stomach than for a woman to lose excess bodyfat around the hips and thighs. The reason for this unjust phenomenon is that fat in the thighs and buttocks is used for long term energy storage, whereas the fat cells in the abdomen are used as a more immediate source of energy.

There is some good news concerning the location of fat in the hips, thighs, and buttocks, however. As frustrating and challenging as it may seem at times, excess body fat in these areas is less threatening to your cardiovascular health than abdominal fat.

Knowing the facts about excess body fat will help you make positive, healthy changes in your lifestyle, which will in turn help you find your own healthy pure energy balance. Yet, most women, especially as they age, will still have some visible body fat, dimples, and bulges. You could spend the rest of your life thinking "If only I had a perfect body, I would be happy" or you can choose to accept and love your body exactly as it is and start fully enjoying your life at this moment, cottage cheese and all.

The amazing thing is that once you surrender to living a truly healthy Pura Vida lifestyle, the energy that you formerly used on "If only" is no longer blocked by negativity and wasted in a relentless pursuit of perfection.

One thing that no one can take away from you is the confidence you gain from feeling good about your healthy body. We have all noticed women who are carrying a little extra weight, yet they appear strong, athletic, and confident, while exuding a joyful, attractive, pure life energy.

When you truly feel good about yourself, knowing that you are taking care of your body and nourishing your spirit, the minor perceived flaws that previously were the focus of much of your energy are no longer as apparent to others since you are not giving them energy by dwelling on them.

By consciously choosing the Pura Vida path and getting in touch with the intuitive side of your nature, you will instinctively want to do the things that are good for you, in turn positively affecting your body's appearance and physical condition.

Applying the helpful Pura Vida stepping stone principles in your daily life will also help you achieve optimal physical and mental health while maintaining a balanced, harmonious state between your mind, body, and spirit. By using the stepping stones, you can also break through the old barriers that may have prevented you from expressing your potential to lead a vibrantly energetic, active lifestyle.

When you make a conscious decision to lead an active lifestyle and make exercise an integral part of your life, you will be gaining more than a firmer, fitter body. Due to improved circulation from cardiovascular improvement, regular exercise increases endorphins, reduces anxiety levels, and decreases muscle tension.

Since aerobic exercise is the most effective way to directly burn excess bodyfat, it is a powerful component in maintaining a strong, physically fit body. Combining weight lifting with aerobic exercise doubles your chances of attaining a body that is not only physically attractive, but healthy and dis-ease free on the inside.

By increasing the strength of your muscles and adding attractive definition with weight training, you will also increase your self-confidence and walk with a noticeable spring in your step that lets people know that you feel good about yourself.

In Chapters 31, 32, and 33, I have included an easy reference guide for muscle anatomy and weight training exercises. In these chapters, you will find a great deal of information specifically related to the fat prone areas of the female body. Of special interest to women is the information in these chapters dealing with the muscles of the buttocks, legs, and hamstrings. I urge you to become familiar with the muscles in these areas so that you can concentrate on working them more effectively.

The weight training exercises discussed in those chapters (specifically for the quads, hamstrings, and adductor and abductor muscles of the thigh) is extremely helpful for women who wish to reduce the appearance of cellulite, as well. In addition, the detailed explanations of various cardiovascular equipment (including treadmills and stationary and recumbent bikes) will provide you with the tools that you need to physically change your body for the better.

Some women seem to be afraid of weight training because they fear that they will become overly muscular. That is difficult to do, however, and does not happen overnight. If you should begin to feel that you are becoming too bulky, you can cut back at any time. The women that you see in magazines with abnormally large, masculine physiques usually work out for several hours a day and use extremely heavy weights. Too often, they also are also endangering their health by taking dangerous steroids.

Women who feel that they are too skinny can benefit tremendously from common sense strength training. Due to metabolic and genetic factors, some women can eat a sufficient amount of calories and still appear to be too thin, and are often unjustly accused of being anorexic. For them, building muscles often also builds self-esteem and confidence.

Of utmost importance to all women is the fact that weight training can help prevent the devastating condition of osteoporosis. While studying anatomy and physiology in Chiropractic College, I remember how exciting it was to discover and learn about the intricate process through which weight bearing exercises help thicken and strengthen the bones by stimulating bone growth. To me, this was another enlightening example of the amazing innate intelligence of the human body adapting to change in a positive way.

This process is somewhat similar in principle to building muscle through resistance in that the body becomes stronger as a reasonable amount of stress is placed on it. Without some physical resistance, our joints and muscles weaken and we are more prone to injury. Since our bodies were designed to be active—walking, jumping, running, and even lifting in moderation—they work best when there is some gentle resistance on the muscles and joints. Resistance naturally builds muscle, and strong muscles lead to a strong foundation.

In addition to strength training, there are some simple exercises you can do at home to target specific areas and increase muscle strength. Below, I have listed a few of my favorite lower body exercises that have stood the test of time. When performed on a regular basis, these exercises really work. You will see accelerated results when you combine them with weight training exercises and a consistent aerobic program.

People frequently ask me what the best type of exercise is. The simple truth is this: the most effective exercises are the ones that you do regularly. Just do something. The secret is pure momentum and consistency. Create your own little arsenal of exercises that you really enjoy doing and that give you the best results.

Always stretch, warm up and cool down with any type of exercise, no matter how simple it may seem. Fortunately, performing the Zoga routine of safe stretching on a consistent basis can make a dramatic difference not only in your energy level but also in your outward appearance.

By elongating muscles and decompressing the spinal column, your posture will naturally improve and your muscles appear to be longer and leaner. I've had many patients tell me that they felt taller after doing these stretches for an extended period of time and I have seen some individual's posture improve so dramatically that they appeared much taller not only to me, but to those who know them well.

In the following chapters, you will find much more specific exercise information and advice. I suggest that you read the entire book for important information about muscle anatomy and injury prevention, in order to gain a broader perspective on the positive benefits of exercise, before significantly altering your current exercise program. You will also find detailed information about the importance of aerobic exercise in burning fat that may dramatically change the way you view exercising for weight loss.

Regarding both floor exercises and strength training exercises, the amount of repetitions (reps) and sets (group of repetitions) that you should do for each exercise varies, depending on your goals, current condition, and how strenuous you find the exercise.

In general, with higher reps (ten or twelve), you will gain more muscle definition. If you can only do five or six reps when you first begin, do not push yourself. Return to your touchstone, the first stepping stone, and listen to the innate wisdom of your body.

As you integrate these exercises into your daily lifestyle, keep in mind that resistance is the major factor that causes your muscles to grow stronger. Much like the resistance you encounter along the path in your everyday life, placing resistance on your muscles makes them stronger and better prepared for the next challenge facing you, whether it be moving furniture or working long hours on too little sleep.

For optimal results, concentrate and focus as you perform these exercises and remember that slow, controlled movements offer continuous resistance against the targeted muscles, resulting in increased strength, tone, and definition.

Listed below are a few powerful, tried and true exercises that will help you build strong muscles in your legs, buttocks, and hip region, and add attractive definition to your entire lower body. These exercises are safe and effective when performed correctly and can be done at home, in a hotel room, or even in the great outdoors.

PELVIC RAISES:

This exercise may look a little awkward but it is especially good for strengthening the muscles of the lower back, buttocks and hamstrings. To perform the pelvic raise, lie face up on the floor with your knees bent considerably, feet flat on the floor, and your hands to your sides.

Then, slowly raise your lower back and hips off the floor to a comfortable position. Concentrate on squeezing your buttocks while raising your hips to the highest comfortable point. Next, hold this position and squeeze hard for at least four or five seconds.

Slowly lower your hips back down to the starting point, breathing deeply throughout the exercise, and then rest for a few seconds and repeat. Focus mainly on contracting and relaxing the buttock muscles. This exercise is particularly good to do if you sit frequently, since it isolates the often neglected muscles of the backside, and helps strengthen the lower back.

SIT BACK SQUATS:

This exercise is very effective and much easier on the knees than the more traditional plie squats, in which the feet are turned outward, possibly stressing the soft tissue of the knee joint. In addition, sit back squats do not involve a compressive force on the spine, but rather focus the workload on the hips and buttocks.

To perform this powerful exercise, you need only your bodyweight and something to hold onto, such as a fixed, upright pole or beam. Stand with the beam in front of you, and place your feet on either side of the beam, extending your toes a few inches in front of it.

Grab onto the beam with your hands. Slowly lower your body as if you were sitting in a straight back chair. You may need to slightly adjust the placement of your feet so that at the bottom of the exercise, your back, knees, and hips are all at right angles to each other. At the bottom of the exercise, your thighs should be parallel with the floor, your back straight, and you should be pressing your weight into your heels.

Hold this sit-back position for a few seconds before beginning to raise your body back up. Your hands should remain stationary throughout the exercise. To keep the resistance constant, raise your body only halfway up, maintaining proper posture throughout the movement.

Do not stand up completely or lock your knees at the top of the exercise. Avoid resting too long between reps. When the sit back squat exercise is done properly, not only will you be firming your buttock muscles and the quad muscles in the front of your legs, but you will also work the muscles of the inner thigh region.

A variation of this exercise which I like to call the sliding squat can be done with your back against a wall. To begin the sliding squat, stand comfortably in front of a wall with your feet placed eight to twelve inches in front of the wall.

With your arms crossed in front of you, begin slowly sliding down the wall, keeping your upper back pressed against it. You may find it necessary to reposition your feet as you gradually lower your body down until you end in a position where your thighs are parallel with the floor. Hold this position for a few seconds before sliding back up the wall.

Avoid locking your knees or straightening your legs at the top of the exercise. In either version of this exercise, resistance is crucial for challenging the muscles and causing them to become stronger.

KICK UPS:

This exercise also isolates the muscles of the buttocks and hamstrings. To perform this powerful exercise, kneel on a carpet or mat on all fours, with your forearms and elbows resting on the floor. You may find it necessary to avoid this position and particular exercise if you have knee or back problems.

With the knee bent, raise your right leg toward the ceiling and press through the heel, as if you were kicking open a trap door in the ceiling. Hold and squeeze the right buttocks for a few seconds, then relax by lowering the leg back to the starting position.

Repeat this motion, concentrating on contracting the muscles of the buttocks and the back of the thighs. Repeat with the left leg. Be careful not to hyperextend or arch your back excessively while performing this exercise. In this Kick-up exercise, intensity and concentration make all the difference. You may also add a small, pulsing type motion at the top of the upward movement that results in added definition.

PRONE LEG RAISES:

Another excellent backside strengthener that is especially good for the hamstrings, lower back, and buttocks muscles is the prone leg raise exercise. Begin this exercise by lying on your stomach with your arms folded under your chin. Then, slowly lift one outstretched leg toward the ceiling, being very careful not to lift your leg too high.

Hold your leg up while squeezing your buttocks for a few seconds in this position. Keep your pelvis flat on the floor. Slowly lower that leg and repeat the exercise with the opposite leg.

Concentrate on isolating the buttock and leg muscles and keeping the leg fairly straight without locking the knee. Do not force the leg to go higher into an uncomfortable position. It is more important to keep the leg extended and focus on the muscles contracting and relaxing as you perform this exercise.

WALKING LUNGES:

Sometimes called traveling lunges, walking lunges are one of the most effective exercises for strengthening the lower body muscles, including the buttocks, thighs and hip area. You will quickly see results with this awesome exercise, including a lifting and tightening of the buttocks muscles and added definition of the thigh muscles. If you have equilibrium or knee problems, however, this may not be the ideal exercise for you.

To begin this exercise, find a long, open area of floor space in which you can take at least six or eight long steps. You may either place your hands on your waist or perform the exercise with dumbbells at your sides. I have found that using hand weights helps me maintain my balance while doing lunges, and I also see more visible results when I increase the amount of weight used, thereby increasing resistance on the leg muscles.

You may, however, choose to perform the exercise without dumbbells until you feel comfortable with the movement. If you choose to use dumbbells, I suggest starting out with light weights. For example, start out using three to five pound dumbbells and then gradually increase the amount of weight as you gain experience and build strength in your leg muscles.

Maintaining proper posture while contracting your stomach muscles for added support is crucial to performing walking lunges. Stand tall with your toes and eyes pointed straight ahead and your feet shoulder width apart. Begin lunging by taking a giant step forward with your right leg. It is helpful to perform this exercise in front of a mirror so that you can see if your foot, ankle, and knee are properly aligned when viewed from the side.

When this exercise is performed properly, your right knee should not extend over the toe of your right foot after you have stepped forward. When viewed from the side, your knee should be directly in line over, or slightly behind, your ankle joint.

At the bottom of the lunge, your left knee should come close to the floor but not touch it. You should feel a gentle stretch in your left leg at this point. Hold this position for a few seconds, then raise your body and take a slow, controlled step with your left leg without pausing in the standing position. Steadily continue lunging forward, pausing only when necessary for balance.

Travel in a straight line, focusing on each movement and concentrating on contracting your leg and buttock muscles. When you have reached the end of your walking area, turn around, rest for a few seconds, and continue lunging toward your starting position. With each step, visualize yourself becoming stronger, steadier, and more confident.

If you do not have adequate floor space, you may prefer to do the stationary version of the lunge. Keep the same precautions in mind, not allowing the knee to extend over the foot, and maintaining proper posture.

Lunge forward with one leg at a time, holding weights if you prefer. The knee of the leg that is not moving forward (the back leg) should come close to, but not touch the floor at the bottom of this exercise.

Return to the starting position with both feet together and repeat the lunges with the same leg. Use high reps if your goal is definition and toning, and lower reps and more weight for increased muscle size. Repeat this process with the other leg, taking sufficient time to rest between sets.

Most of the exercises listed above involve some type of squeezing and holding of the muscles, which helps isometrically contract the involved muscle and results in added definition. Also utilizing the same principle, any time you find yourself standing in one spot for an extended period of time, take advantage of the opportunity to isometrically contract your calf, stomach, leg, and buttocks muscles. Not only does this practice improve circulation, which can help varicose veins, but it also helps firm the muscles and makes you consciously aware of the muscles of your lower body.

If you are tired of feeling bad about yourself, it is time to something about it. Begin consistently performing some simple exercises that work for you. Do not wait until that magical day when all the conditions are perfect and you begin a program "For good this time."

Adopting an active, healthy lifestyle begins with an active mindset and positive attitude. Tell yourself that it is okay to play without a lot of rules and regulations; to simply move for the sake of movement. Even if you were not very active or athletic when you were younger, you can be more energetic and vibrant starting right now!

Chase your kids or pets around the yard, challenge your walking partner to an impulsive dash to a distant tree, or try your hand at a new sport or outdoor activity that keeps you moving. Apply what you have learned thus far along your Pura Vida journey in your everyday life, keeping in mind that nothing has more power over your body than your mind.

Use that power to visualize yourself leading an active, healthy, fun lifestyle and allow that vision to be reflected in your personality, attitude, and relationships. Your true power and pure energy comes from within. Do not keep it hidden. Let it out and be the zesty, young at heart, fun-loving person that you truly are.

The Power Of Exercise

Throughout our adventures in Costa Rica, Len and I were blessed with numerous encounters and learning experiences that caused us to look at our definitions of physical activity and fitness in a new light. One such encounter was a particularly humbling, yet enlightening experience.

After hiking for most of the day on a steep, physically challenging path, we stopped to rest on top of a sunny knoll covered with soft green grass.

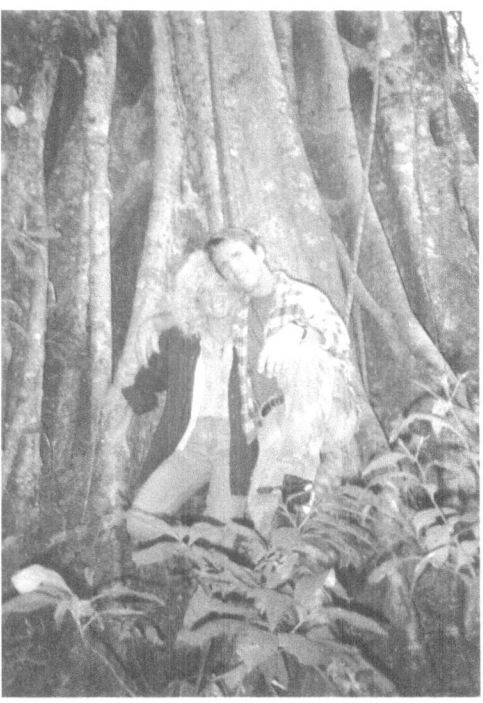

From this vantage point, we could see a powerful *cascada* (waterfall) in the distance, tucked far away in the next mountain range, fading in and out through the misty clouds, moving rapidly across a surreal blue sky.

Our spirits lifted as we watched the soaring flight of a pair of swallow tailed kites, skimming over the rolling, green sea of trees in the lush valley. Recharging our batteries in the sun, we congratulated ourselves on the physical accomplishment of our long, invigorating hike.

Our somewhat smug sense of self-satisfaction was short lived, however, when there, in the middle of nowhere, at the bottom of an impassable, almost vertical road; we spotted a robust looking Tico who must have been at least in his mid-seventies.

With a large pick, he was slowly clearing a trench along the rocky road. As we observed him gradually working his way toward us, we were impressed with his physical endurance, perseverance, and flexibility. A broad, joyful smile spread across his face as he approached us and we began to communicate with him in broken Spanish. His sense of self-worth and peaceful nature were clearly evident in the confident way that he held his body.

He explained that the mystical waterfall we were admiring in the distance belonged to him, as did the large *finca* (farm) surrounding it. He could barely contain his pride as his fist covered his chest and he repeated the words *"Mi finca"* (my farm).

In sharp contrast to his weathered face, his twinkling eyes radiated ceaseless energy and pure life. After exchanging heartfelt "Pura Vidas" we watched him walk away with a youthful spring in his step and a proud smile on his face. His strong, compact body seemed as if it should have belonged to a much younger man.

The enthusiasm and zest with which the farmer tackled his meaningful task of digging ditches serves as a continual source of inspiration to me, especially when I find myself caught up in daily routines or with limited energy to devote to mundane tasks.

Our encounter with the farmer served as a powerful lesson that physical fitness is a relative term that cannot be defined simply by medical charts and laboratory tests. Optimal health includes the joy of living your life in true present time, with an exuberant spring in your step and fresh air circulating through your lungs.

I have found that when I remind myself of truths such as the one we learned from this proud, hard working farmer, it helps me to put my life in perspective. Little life lessons such as this help me to strengthen my resolve to continue on a healthy path, and do whatever I may be doing at that time joyfully, and with a sense of purpose, living fully in the moment.

I was also reminded of the robust farmer and the importance of living life fully in the moment during a trip to San Francisco. In a tiny green oasis, surrounded by the steep streets and busy clamor of this fascinating city, Len and I witnessed a small group of peaceful looking, older Chinese men engaging in another form of meaningful exercise, which, to them, is as important as eating or sleeping. In the dappled, early morning light, these gentle souls were gracefully performing the ancient art of Tai Chi, moving very slowly, yet with unbelievable precision and focus.

Practitioners of this ancient art believe that not only does Tai Chi tone and strengthen muscles and tissues, but also, that the practice supplies life energy and keeps chi circulating throughout the body. In China, it is not unusual to see people of all ages practicing Tai Chi or Qi Gong in parks and in their yards in the morning, moving purposefully and concentrating intently in order to find their center, or chi, which, they believe is actually health itself.

A life filled with maximum energy can only arise from an energetically balanced lifestyle. Since the mind and body coexist in a yin/yang relationship, an energy imbalance in one creates an energy imbalance in the other. One way of balancing your mind and body's energies is through mindful exercise, which engages both mental and physical energy simultaneously.

It seems unfortunate that some people still seem to view exercise as a difficult chore, not as a normal invigorating, energy producing aspect of their every day lives. All too often I hear people say, "I just don't have enough energy to exercise." What many of them do not realize is that the exertion of energy in the right direction creates more pure energy. The very thing that many people believe takes energy is the same thing that can produce it.

The most popular reason most of us (myself included) have for not exercising is lack of time. Yet, have you ever noticed that if you really want to find the time to do something, it somehow makes its way into your schedule? It is basically a matter of making exercise a very high priority in your life; a *want to* or *have to* rather than a *should* or *need to*.

I firmly believe that the current interest in health and fitness is not simply another passing trend or fad. It is a Pura Vida way of life that is here to stay. It appears to me that, as a society, we are rapidly evolving and becoming wiser, fully realizing that regular exercise and a high level of physical activity is a necessary, integral part of a healthy, balanced lifestyle.

What many of us have always held as a core belief is gradually being absorbed into the recommendations (although not necessary the personal lifestyles) of our country's medical and scientific communities. Nearly every doctor in America is finally prescribing exercise.

In fact, the surgeon general's report on physical activity and health finally confirmed what most of us have known all along, that lack of physical exercise is detrimental to your health. The key finding of this report is that people of all ages can improve the quality of their lives through a lifelong practice of moderate physical activity.

In addition, the report concludes that regular physical activity enhances mental health, greatly reduces the risk of dying from coronary heart disease, and also decreases the risk of developing diabetes, hypertension, and colon cancer.

I hope that this recent scientific validation will serve as part of the impetus toward a dramatic shift in health consciousness that focuses on the importance of preventing disease, thereby reducing the need for spending billions of dollars per year on drugs and surgery.

In the past few years, I have been extremely pleased to see the increasing popularity of mind-body exercises such as yoga and Pilates. Every day, more people are living their dream of creating a healthier lifestyle by incorporating exercise and activities into their life, and balancing and strengthening the connection between their body, mind, and soul.

Over the years, I have had the privilege and pleasure of working with numerous elite and world class athletes, as well as countless weekend warriors who work hard and play even harder. Their enthusiasm and commitment have inspired and motivated me to push my own limits and share some of my observations and research with others. Hopefully, some of my experiences will benefit you as you strive to achieve your own unique health and fitness goals.

When I first began researching athletic potential, I was somewhat surprised to find that one of the attributes that sets elite athletes apart has more to do with the mind than with the physical body. Most world-class athletes possess an extraordinary ability to block out all distractions, while concentrating and focusing solely on the present moment and visualizing their future success.

As 2004 Olympic swimmer Natalie Coughlin explains, "The winning secret is not strength, not height, but focus." She states that when she is in the pool, she focuses on whatever technique she is working on that day. There are layer upon layers of things to think about, she says, such as concentrating on building her core muscles so that when she gets tired, her technique does not deteriorate.

Increasing the ability to focus and block out extraneous noise and chatter is a difficult challenge for most of us in today's hyper speed world. When we take time to center ourselves through practices such as creative visualization and meditation, however, we too can accomplish goals that may have previously seemed unattainable.

Self discipline is another common trait among the best of the best athletes in the world. Olympic medalists are masters at disciplining their bodies and minds to achieve optimal results. It is not unusual for athletes training for competition in the Olympics to spend a minimum of six or eight hours a day, six or seven days a week training for their particular event or sport.

Their days usually start early in the morning, when many of us are still sleeping, and are filled not only with training and drills for their specific sport or event, but also devoted to countless hours of conditioning their bodies with practices such as strength and resistance training, plyometrics, stretching, and speed work.

Another area that self discipline is evident in is the nutritional aspect of elite athlete's daily lives. They realize that nutrition and exercise are integrally related and are acutely aware of everything that goes into their bodies. They see quality food as the fuel necessary to provide energy and finely tune their bodies. They drink enormous amounts of pure water and almost always supplement their diets with quality vitamins and minerals containing health promoting substances such as phytochemicals and antioxidants.

Most world class athletes seem to instinctively value the importance of holistic health care and are some of the most open minded people that I have ever encountered. They take responsibility for the state of their own well being and continually educate themselves about health and fitness topics such as exercise physiology, sports nutrition, and biomechanics.

Increasing numbers of elite athletes take advantage of the vast knowledge base and experience of Holistic and Alternative health care providers who treat the entire body and not simply isolated parts. In addition, record numbers of professional athletes utilize the services of alternative practitioners such as massage therapists, yoga and pilates instructors, acupuncturists, and herbalists.

Part of the reason that many of the world's greatest athletes are loyal supporters of natural health care systems stems from the fact that they truly appreciate the specificity of the advice and treatment related to their unique conditions and health and fitness goals.

Fortunately, you don't have to be an elite athlete to benefit from the subjects listed above. With just a little extra focus, awareness, and self discipline, most of us can discover reserves of confidence and inner strength within ourselves that motivate and inspire us to be the best that we can be.

It is my hope that reading the following facts will provide you with added motivation to make consistent exercise and physical activity an integral part of your Pura Vida journey. Keep the facts below in mind as you move forward through the concrete jungle, using your inner wisdom as a practical tool, like a powerful machete, removing any obstacles lying in the way of your path of optimal health.

Since cardiovascular disease is destroying the lives and health of so many of our loved ones today, it is crucial for us all to remember that regular exercise can help raise the good HDLs and lower the bad LDLs, which reduces the risk of deadly cardiovascular disease.

Also, exercise and physical activity improve the overall function of the cardiovascular system, particularly the pumping action of the heart muscle. This is especially important for people over age thirty, because it is normally at this age that the blood pumping capacity of the heart muscle begins to gradually decline. Perhaps if the heart were a more visible muscle, such as the arms or abdominal muscles, we would pay more attention to keeping it in shape.

Also, as noted in the Surgeon General's report, exercise can reduce the risk of another killer disease, colon cancer, by aiding in proper elimination of food through the digestive system. Some more good news to keep in mind is that some of the people who suffer from both the inflammatory type of arthritis (rheumatoid) and the degenerative type (osteoarthritis) can benefit greatly from certain types of moderate exercise.

Several types of cancer, such as breast, colon, and kidney, have been linked to obesity. Since exercise is an integral part of combating obesity, it can help reduce the risk of these cancers. Your body was designed to function most efficiently when your activity level is high. Everything simply works better. As recent research indicates, being inactive and unfit is nearly as significant a risk factor for death as smoking.

When combined with the right foods from the correct sources, regular aerobic exercise has specific health promoting benefits. The term aerobic literally means in the presence of oxygen. Aerobic exercise include activities such as walking, running, biking, and other exercises which cause you to breathe deeply and with added effort.

Sufficient aerobic activity is necessary to supply oxygen to the body so that it can metabolize or burn fat. Regular aerobic exercise also increases the level of calorie consuming enzymes inside the muscle. Aerobic exercise does more that just burn calories, however. Aerobic exercise actually changes the body's chemistry making it easier to burn fat, rather than simply store it.

Not only does physical activity raise your metabolic rate and increase your amount of metabolically active muscle tissue, but physical activity also speeds up vascular and lymphatic flow. All of the systems of your magnificent body, including the nervous, digestive, circulatory, and respiratory systems, simply function more efficiently when you make exercise a regular part of your Pura Vida lifestyle.

Len and I can personally vouch for the positive effects that regular exercise and activity have on our relationships—with each other and also with family and friends. Quite honestly, we have found that exercising and working out together has enriched our relationship on many different levels, including the intimate and spiritual aspects of our daily lives.

Long before there was a scientific name for things such as HDL's and fat burning enzymes, the energetic trail blazers of the original Pura Vida Path were naturally getting plenty of exercise and physical activity in their daily lives.

They believed so passionately in movement that they placed not one, but four Stepping stones along your path that are involved with making exercise and physical activity an integral part of your daily lifestyle. Reaching the next rewarding stepping stone along your Pura Vida Odyssey requires patience, persistence, and mental flexibility.

To reach this point in your journey you must grab the twisted vines along the path for support and pull yourself up using only the strength of your own muscles. Once again, no one else can do this for you. After taking a short, but powerful leap upward, you confidently place your feet on a solid, wide ledge that is actually composed of several progressive levels of similar helpful stepping stones.

The twelfth stepping stone is the first of four related to exercise and draws heavily on the knowledge gained from two previous important stepping stones. By tying together the principles of momentum (Stepping Stone # 8) and Pure Energy Balance (Stepping Stone # 5), your Pura Vida guides placed this next crucial stepping stone at precisely the right point along the path.

Stepping Stone # 12: *Taking time to make exercise and physical activity a consistent, integral part of your high-energy lifestyle is the twelfth Stepping stone along your path.*

You have progressed thus far along your journey to this awe-inspiring height by fully understanding the principle of energy balance. You realize that by taking in quality energy, not only nutritionally but psychologically, spiritually, creatively, and socially, (your energy input) you can create high quality energy output for sustaining a physically, mentally, and spiritually fulfilling and balanced life.

You also realize that maintaining a healthy momentum by consistently engaging in exercise and physical activity is a natural part of this circular, free flow of energy. You believe that exercise not only uses high quality energy but also produces it. You are encouraged and motivated to exercise by always keeping in mind the multitude of positive, health related benefits of regular exercise and physical activity.

You listen to the innate wisdom of your body and are fully aware of the importance of preventing disease, not simply waiting until problems occur to make your health a high priority. Keep up the good work. You are on the right path.

Feeling Stronger Every Day

As you stand confidently on the lower portion of the rock ledge formed by the twelfth stepping stone, seize the moment, and take time to soak up the expansive view from this new perspective. Remember that your true vision extends as far as your mind can see, as you use the awesome power of creative visualization to picture yourself becoming stronger and healthier.

Just as the most fulfilling and lasting rewards come from fully enjoying and appreciating each step of the Pure Life journey rather than hurrying toward a final destination, the rewards and benefits of exercise and movement should be fully enjoyed and appreciated as you are engaging in them.

Acquiring the maximum energy that accompanies a balanced life takes place on an ongoing daily basis rather than as a result of reaching one specific goal or certain destination. In order to permanently integrate physical activity and exercise into your day-to-day lifestyle, you may need to spend some time experimenting to find the unique combination of sports, exercise, or activities that are best for you.

To increase the odds of making exercise and movement a permanent part of your Pura Vida lifestyle, it is imperative that you choose an exercise or combination of exercises that you truly enjoy doing, so much so that you actually look forward to the next time. We are all unique individuals who tap into a different type of energy and level of awareness when we find the combination of exercises, sports, or activities that is uniquely right for us. Much like the mental and spiritual aspects of your steadily evolving lifestyle, this combination may vary from day to day, or change entirely as you evolve and continue along the path of personal growth.

Naturally, many of us have physical limitations. As with everything else in our lives, we learn to work within our safe boundaries and make the most of what we do have. Observing amazing accomplishments such as those of highly skilled athletes participating in sports from their wheelchairs or runners sprinting on artificial limbs, serves as an excellent reminder to us all, however, that certain limitations can be adapted to and overcome.

By practicing what you learned from the first stepping stone, tuning in to the innate intelligence of your body, you will receive valuable warning signs and information about the healthy limits of your body. By paying attention to this information, you will eventually be able to distinguish between signs such as joint pain versus muscle soreness, or proper stretching versus muscle tearing.

To obtain an accurate picture of your specific physical condition and current fitness level, you should obtain a thorough physical exam from the health care practitioner of your choice before starting any strenuous exercise program. Knowing exactly what condition your heart, respiratory system, spine, and joints are in is especially important when you are just beginning to condition your body with various types of aerobic exercise.

If exercise is only a faint memory to you, it is very important that you start out slowly and pace yourself. If you begin by over-exerting yourself, not only do you risk injury, but also you will probably not look forward to exercising again, and consequently, exercise will quickly move closer to the bottom of your priority list.

A health club or gym membership is often one of the best investments that many people can make in their health. Not only do most health clubs have a wide variety of strength training and cardiovascular equipment, Certified Personal Trainers, childcare, aerobics, Yoga, Pilates, and other fun and interesting classes, but they also can provide a strong sense of camaraderie and social support.

One of the advantages of exercising in a gym or health club environment is that you are there for one specific reason, and unlike working out at home, you are less likely to be distracted by telephones, television, the refrigerator, household chores, family, friends, and visitors.

Creating a home gym may be the best choice for you, however, if you are a self-motivated, disciplined person. You can save a considerable amount of time not having to commute to the gym and wait in line for machines.

Although we have thoroughly enjoyed working out in gyms for most of our adult lives, several years ago Len and I decided to create a home gym, mainly due to time and distance restrictions. Over the years, we have maintained gym memberships but now have the option of working out at home on days when traffic and time constraints are prohibitive. By investing in home equipment, gradually adding one piece at a time, we have created a private, convenient spot where we spend quality time together exercising our bodies and minds.

The only disadvantage we have found with this arrangement is that we do not have enough room for as wide of a variety of machines and equipment as a well-equipped public gym. Consequently we have become a little more creative and make efficient use of what we do have.

Whether you belong to a health club or work out at home, the bottom line is that you can own the most expensive, high tech equipment in the world, and it does you no good whatsoever unless you consistently use it. Some people can maintain healthy, strong physiques with nothing but a few dumbbells or the weight of their own bodies, and plenty of self discipline and sheer determination.

My favorite place to work out is still the great outdoors, taking full advantage of the tenth Stepping stone by spending quality time connecting with nature and concentrating on practicing healthy deep breathing in the fresh air.

Some of my happiest, most vivid memories involve some form of exercise or physical activity, whether swimming in sparkling aquamarine waters, exploring exciting uncharted territory on foot, bikes, or skates, or simply walking through rustling autumn leaves on a soul warming, fall day. Perhaps you also share similar unforgettable memories associated with being in nature and moving your body, breathing deeply, and living life to its fullest potential.

When you come to the end of your days on this earth, it is these memories that you will longingly look back on, possibly wishing that you still had the strength or good health to simply run, walk, climb, or play sports. As our treasured senior friends always tell us "Enjoy life while you can!" Take their advice, seize the moment, and get out there and create some memories.

If engaging in exercise, athletics, and other physical activities is somewhat unexplored territory to you, you may want to simply get your feet wet and test the waters gradually rather than jumping in head first. Do not be disappointed if the fantastic benefits of consistent exercise and physical activity that I have been discussing do not manifest themselves immediately. It may take your body some time to adjust to a more active lifestyle, especially if all it is accustomed to is wearing a path from the television to the couch to the refrigerator.

People often tell me, "I'll give it a couple of weeks" expecting immediate results, even though it may have taken them years to get out of shape. You may not develop extra energy and a firmer body after just a few workouts. The fact that you do not see the transformation taking place on the outside does not mean that your body is not changing for the better on the inside, however.

As you have already discovered, utilizing the awesome power of your mind to focus your energy on a certain outcome increases the odds that it will happen. As top professional, Olympic, and world-class athletes are finding, getting into the right mental shape is as important as physical conditioning. The U.S. Track and Field team believes so firmly in the power of the mind that they work with a team of psychologists year-round and during the Olympics.

Whether you are a certified couch potato or a professional athlete, there lies an extraordinary potential within you. The power of your own energy is limited only by the amount of time and effort you are willing to devote to developing it. By strengthening your physical body through the practice of regular exercise, you are also strengthening your mind and spirit, and building up your energy reserves for future use as well.

Paying special attention to your breathing and pulse rate are two good ways to help further connect your mind and body during exercise. Your heart and lungs are truly amazing organs that can supply you with valuable information about the intricate inner workings of your physical body.

One of the most important things to remember when performing any type of exercise is to keep your heart rate (the rate or speed at which your heart beats) within a safe zone. This is especially important if you are just beginning to break free from the bonds of an inactive lifestyle.

To achieve maximum cardiovascular benefits from aerobic exercise, you will want to establish your own unique target heart rate range. (In reading the following, keep in mind that the word rate pertains to speed and the word range involves an upper and lower limit).

Also, please keep in mind that although the following explanation and details of establishing your safe target heart rate are important, the information is a bit complicated. Fortunately, it doesn't have to be memorized and assimilated at this moment if it creates a stumbling block in your Pura Vida momentum. You can always skim over it, bookmark and return to this page when you are ready to apply the principle.

It is important that you exercise within your target heart rate range, not only to gain maximum benefit, but to avoid overexertion. The condition of everyone's cardiovascular system is different, based on many variables including age, physical condition, and current exercise level, so the Target Heart Rate is only an estimate. It does, however, represent a convenient rule of thumb.

To check your pulse, hold one palm face up. With the first two fingers of your other hand, lightly press downward on your outer wrist. Do not use your thumb to check your pulse. Adjust the position of your fingers until you feel the strongest pulse. Count the beats in fifteen seconds and multiply by four (or thirty seconds and multiply by two) to give you your pulse rate for one minute.

A normal resting pulse rate is somewhere around sixty to ninety beats per minute. It is sometimes more convenient to check your pulse in the large artery in your neck with your fingertips as you exercise. You can check either side, but must be careful to never occlude both arteries in your neck at the same time.

As you are checking your pulse, take a moment to visualize the life giving, oxygenated blood flowing through the elaborate web of arteries and veins in your circulatory system with every beat of your heart. Picture your powerful heart muscle pumping healthy blood throughout its chambers with precision timing and utmost efficiency.

You may find it interesting to check your pulse at different times of the day, and in different states of emotion to see what is a normal pulse rate for you. During strenuous aerobic exercise, I often check my pulse at regular intervals to make sure that I am exercising within safe boundaries and not placing undue stress on my heart.

Now, it gets a little more complicated. Now that you are familiar with taking your pulse, you will want to learn how to calculate your safe target heart rate range. Your target heart rate (THR) range is between 65–85% of your maximum heart rate, depending on your current fitness level, with 70% being the average for the intermediate level.

If you are just beginning an exercise program, you should start by working toward the low end of the range, gradually working your way toward the higher end over time. Exercising at the upper end of this range is only recommended for people who are already well conditioned. For these people, the heart is effectively but safely stressed at this level.

Finding your THR range is really not as complicated as it may seem. As the name implies, your maximum heart rate is the rate or speed at which your heart is unable to pump efficiently any faster.

To begin your target heart rate calculations, simply subtract your age from 220 to obtain your maximum heart rate. Then multiply this number by .65 and .85 to find the lower and upper limits of your THR.

For example, if you are thirty years old and just beginning an exercise program, this is how you would calculate your target heart rate range: 220 minus 30 (your age) equals 190, which would be your maximum heart rate.

Now, to find the safe target heart rate range, you would multiply 190 by .65 (which equals 123) to establish the lower end of your THR (target heart rate) range. Then you would multiply 190 by .85 (which equals 161) to establish the upper end of your specific THR range.

This means that, as a beginner, you should aim to reach and maintain the lower level of 123 beats per minute or slightly higher, for the duration of your aerobic workout, stopping periodically to monitor your pulse rate. Over time, you should gradually progress toward the upper level of your THR range. If you have consulted a qualified health care provider about your exercise program, be sure to follow his or her advice concerning your suggested target heart rate.

Perhaps most importantly, use the first powerful Stepping Stone as a touchstone and listen to the warning signals from your body when engaging in any form of aerobic exercise. When your heart and lungs tell you that you are pushing too hard or have had enough, pay attention to the innate intelligence of your magnificent body.

Stretching For Health

Now that you have broken new ground and committed to making exercise and physical activity an integral part of your high energy lifestyle (Stepping Stone #12) you are ready for what just may be my personal favorite stepping stone. Stepping Stone #13 lies at the base of a resilient, yet tall and straight tree growing out of a rocky ledge along your path. Although the tree has been hammered and blasted by gale force winds and other inclement weather, it has never snapped and broken, because its design incorporates the principle of flexible strength.

Stepping Stone #13: *Include a regular program of stretching into your daily lifestyle.* This powerful yet simple stepping stone has changed my life for the better and benefited me in so many ways that it would be hard to list them all here. I am confident that it can make a positive difference in your life as well.

Before I introduce you to the next helpful Pura Vida lifestyle tool, I'd like to share something with you that may have a direct impact on your life. Throughout my entire childhood and adult years, I have always been what I think of as a truth seeker. The specific areas that have consistently held my interest over the years are those related to holistic health and natural fitness.

My winding life path lead me to become a Chiropractor at a young age and help thousands of individuals with neck and back pain and a variety of other symptoms and conditions. I am extremely grateful for my experiences as a DC and am proud to be part of a forward thinking profession that has helped bring the benefits of holistic and natural health care into the mainstream—one patient at a time. I'm a firm believer in the gradual corrective process of adjusting or manipulating the spine in order to create a more healthy nervous system and structural foundation.

The practice of chiropractic is a full time job and for a truly dedicated practitioner, there is often little time left at the end of the day for a balanced personal life. In all honesty, there were many times in my professional life that I felt a bit hypocritical, lecturing my patients about subjects such as stress reduction, prioritizing and taking time for yourself. As someone who truly enjoys sharing information and advice with others, I often felt frustrated by time constraints and often found myself wishing I had more time to educate my patients about self care.

My choice to follow the path of a teacher and educator was a deliberate, conscious choice that came as a surprise to many. As a student, I spent much of my life soaking up information and research that was valuable to me and others with similar interests and goals. Before there were insightful books such as *The Purpose Driven Life*, I felt strongly that part of my reason for being on the planet was to share what I have learned with others on a broad scale.

The information that follows below is the cumulative result of more than twenty years of exploring and researching a subject that is near and dear to my heart. Based on my experience, I truly believe that if everyone were to follow this simple practice on a daily basis, the world would be a little less stressful and a lot less painful and rigid place. I'm sure that many teachers of various techniques, methods, and practices believe the same thing, and on same level perhaps we are all correct in our thinking and intent.

So, what could possibly be so powerful and life changing that I would dedicate such a large chunk of my life and energy to it? A simple, safe, and effective daily stretching program that I have developed called Zoga. As I mentioned earlier, you can find out much more about Zoga by visiting www.pure-life.com and clicking on the Zoga link.

Basically what I have done is take my favorite stretching exercises from various disciplines such as therapeutic and rehabilitative stretching, yoga, and other health care systems such as chiropractic and combined them in an easy to perform, flowing series of standing and mat stretches.

Part of my motivation for creating the Zoga method of safe stretching was that I was never fully satisfied with the stretching exercises that were available as a reference to my patients in the past. Although there are literally hundreds of more stretches that are both safe and effective, these are the ones that made my final cut for the general population and can be done by most individuals with relatively good health and fairly normal range of motion.

I'm a big fan of Yoga and have seen or heard of this ancient practice literally changing the bodies, minds, and souls of countless individuals, but in all honesty, Yoga isn't for everyone. I've tried it many times and liked it, but I always come back to my simple, tried and true Zoga routine, as have many of the individuals who I have taught the Zoga method. Their enthusiastic testimonials and visible improvements are what has kept me going over the years.

If you are currently practicing Yoga or Pilates on a regular basis and have no difficulties or discomfort, keep up the good work! Adding Zoga to your existing practice can only serve to help you achieve more of the positive results that you strive for.

So, what can this simple practice do for you? When performed on a daily basis, this powerful, flowing series of exercises will increase joint flexibility and muscle strength, as well as tone muscles, relieve joint pain, improve posture, and reduce stress.

In addition, these low-impact stretches elongate muscles and decompress joints while taking them through their normal ranges of motion. Please notice that I said normal ranges of motion. With these stretches, you won't be twisting your body like a pretzel or pushing it past any limits that don't feel right for you.

Zoga is easy to learn and takes only ten to fifteen minutes a day. All you need is a thick, cushioned mat. You can use a thin yoga mat if the carpet you are lying on is thickly padded. Take off your shoes and belts and wear comfortable, loose clothing that allows you to move and stretch easily. The routine is divided into two parts: Part One (Sets 1–6) is the Standing Portion. Part Two (Sets 7–10) is the Mat Portion (Floor exercises).

You should perform the routine at least once a day, any time of day. Some people find that doing Zoga twice a day, in the morning and evening works best for them. You can also do specific exercises throughout your day if you choose. Be sure to listen to your body and take your time. Don't forget to breathe!

You will achieve optimal results if you do the routine in front of a full length mirror, but it isn't absolutely necessary to have one. When you first learn the routine, it helps to watch yourself moving in a mirror to monitor your progress. As you become more familiar with the exercises you may choose to close your eyes to increase your focus during some of the easier stretches.

I've found it extremely helpful to take the time to create a peaceful area to do your daily stretches. You don't need a great deal of floor space so you can do your routine just about anywhere, even when you are traveling. Try to minimize interruptions. This is your time, so turn off the phone ringer and lock the door if possible.

Listen to relaxing and soothing music if you wish. You may obtain better results if you listen to the same music each time you do your Zoga routine. Repeating the same routine daily helps reinforce neural pathways and signals your body to relax even more deeply.

Although the word routine sometimes has negative associations, in this instance it is a very positive thing because each time you move through the exercises, it becomes more natural for you and you are able to relax deeper and deeper without having to think about what comes next.

Practicing deep breathing while performing the exercises is crucial. You'll see faster results when you breathe deeply from your stomach and you will be decreasing the negative effects of stress on your body as well.

Hold stretches for as long as you are comfortable, the slower the better. Once you have learned the routine, try to remember what exercise comes next, so one exercise flows smoothly into the next. Don't give up. You can memorize this routine and make it your own. The more you do it, the easier it gets and the more comfortable your body becomes going through the ranges of motion.

If you are looking for a simple stretching routine that works all parts of your body quickly, then please take some time to visit pure-life.com and begin learning all about this simple, life changing practice at your convenience. You might just become a believer and join the grassroots Zoga Revolution!

Once you are familiar with the Zoga Routine, you will always have an arsenal of safe and effective stretches to choose from before engaging in sports, weight training and other athletic pursuits as well.

Always take the time to stretch and elongate the muscles, warm up the joints, and work on increasing flexibility before exercising. The positive effects you will gain in your workout and daily activities are well worth the time and effort and will help reduce the negative effects of stress and gravity on your body.

Improper stretching and insufficient time spent warming up can result in serious soft tissue damage, involving muscles, tendons, and ligaments, especially for people with a hurry up and get it over with philosophy concerning exercise.

To prevent unnecessary, frustrating delays, a regular stretching routine should be an integral part of any exercise program. You should always warm up prior to exercise, and cool down afterward in order to prevent injury. Stretches should be done slowly and gently, taken to a comfortable position, and held steadily.

Soft tissue strain or sprain can sometimes set you back for months in your exercise program. One of the worst mistakes that many people make is to overstretch a body part, forcing it to the point of pain, or to use bouncy, jerky motions while stretching.

Although the word sprain is often used generically to describe different types of injury to a joint, it actually has a more specific meaning. A sprain involves the tearing of a ligament, which is the connective tissue that holds two bones together.

Muscle strain, (involving muscles and their tendons) will often occur at the same time as a sprain, especially with ankle sprains. Here is a helpful little pneumonic: I remember the difference between strains and sprains by linking the letter 't' in the word tendon to the letter 't' in the word strain.

Often, when you are pressed for time, skipping before and after stretching seems like the easiest way to add minutes to your workout. Although you may not notice any side effects or immediate injury from inadequate stretching, there is always an adverse effect.

Inadequate stretching can result in minute tears or ruptures of individual muscle fibers, which are not always immediately noticeable. Once the soft tissue is torn, it loses some of its elasticity, and becomes a weak spot that is prone to future injury.

The most important thing to remember with all stretches is to perform them slowly, gently, and carefully for maximum results. A few extra minutes spent stretching properly can save you weeks, even months, of down time in the long run.

Make the most of your stretching time by practicing deep breathing, creative visualization, and mentally preparing yourself for the upcoming exercise. Try not to let life pass you by too fast. Take your own sweet tranquilo time and fully enjoy all of the life changing benefits of flexible strength.

Exercising Aerobically

Before you can fully enjoy the magnificent, panoramic Pura Vida view from another, even higher level of the multi-tiered exercise ledge, it helps to have fully integrated what you have learned from the third, deep breathing stepping stone into your daily lifestyle.

During exercise, your body works harder than it is accustomed to working, and your muscles demand more oxygen. The capacity of your lungs increases and your heart becomes stronger and larger as it works to pump life sustaining, oxygen-rich blood through the arteries.

The only type of exercise that directly burns bodyfat is aerobic (with oxygen) exercise because, for fat to be burned, oxygen must be present. During aerobic exercises such as running or swimming, the heart and lungs are able to supply the muscles with oxygen at a continuous, fairly strenuous pace. Conversely, anaerobic (without oxygen) exercises, such as weight lifting, involve sudden bursts of strenuous activity lasting less than ten seconds.

The more aerobically fit your body is, the more efficiently it uses oxygen during exercise. Consistent aerobic exercise conditions and strengthens the heart muscle, respiratory system, and also the musculoskeletal system. Aerobic conditioning results in more efficient function during any sustained physical activity that you engage in, whether it is shoveling snow, raking leaves, or playing tennis.

The wise designers of the Pura Vida path instinctively incorporated natural forms of aerobic exercise in their everyday lives. Consequently, they had little difficulty placing the next irreplaceable sturdy rock into the ledge formed by the four interlocking exercise related stepping stones.

Stepping Stone #14: *Include consistent aerobic exercise in your everyday Pura Vida Lifestyle for optimal health, energy, and stamina.*

As your awareness increases, you will find your own unique way of integrating the lessons learned from each of the Pura Vida Stepping Stones into your daily life. You will also find that when you make positive changes in order to become healthier, there are usually unexpected, pleasantly surprising benefits and rewards in other aspects of your daily life.

Such is the case with the added benefit of a more attractive appearance of your outer body when you perform consistent aerobic exercise to increase the strength and health of your inner body and internal organs, such as the heart and lungs.

The quickest way to obtain a firm body with some attractive muscular definition is to combine regular aerobic exercise with strength training. This powerful combination doubles the fat burning effect, directly through aerobic exercise and indirectly by increasing lean muscle mass through weight training.

To obtain optimal whole body aerobic benefits, the exercise should involve the large muscles of the legs and buttocks and should demand a steady, uninterrupted output from your muscles. Involving the large muscles of your lower body results in more of a whole body, systemic effect because the large, broad muscles in the buttocks and the front and back of the upper leg require more oxygen than the smaller, thinner muscles of the arms, for example.

Patients and friends frequently ask me about the effectiveness of aerobic exercise machines that they see advertised on television. Some machines are more effective than others, however, the simple truth is, no machine is going to get you in shape unless you use it consistently. You are the only one who can do that. Regardless of what you pay for a piece of exercise equipment, you will only get out of it what you put into it.

Here are a few key points to remember about some of the more popular machines designed to maximize your aerobic potential.

STATIONARY BIKES:

Stationary or recumbent bicycles are an excellent low impact starting point for those just beginning aerobic exercise. The recumbent stationary bicycles found in most gyms allow you to sit in a comfortable position with your legs stretched out in front of you while you pedal. Make sure that the seat is adjusted properly on the stationary upright or recumbent bike. When you sit on the bicycle, there should be a slight bend in the knee of your extended leg.

The primary muscles worked on upright and recumbent stationary bikes are your quadriceps muscles in the front of your thighs. Although your upper body gets little or no workout, there is minimal weight bearing pressure on the knees and ankles with an adjustable level of pedaling resistance. It is easy to build up your cardiovascular time quickly on a stationary bike, gradually progressing to longer aerobic sessions, which increase your fat burning potential.

One convenient thing about stationary bikes is that it is fairly easy to read while using them, possibly killing two birds with one stone in your busy day. Len and I have a recumbent bike in front of our television at home and find it very effective for cardiovascular conditioning and body fat loss when used on a consistent basis.

TREADMILL:

Treadmills work mostly the muscles of the legs and buttocks and are an efficient tool for cardiovascular conditioning. They are effective for all levels; from beginning exercisers who wish to start out slowly and gradually improve their speed and endurance, to advanced exercisers who are seeking a rigorous fat burning and cardiovascular exercise.

It is extremely important to wear a shoe with plenty of cushioning for shock absorption, especially if you plan to jog or run. I cannot stress this point enough. I've seen several people suffer needless injuries on the treadmill simply because they wore improper or worn out athletic shoes.

Get the most benefit you can out of the treadmill by gradually raising the incline upward. This will give the gluteal muscles more of a workout, and increase cardiovascular conditioning. If you have hip or joint problems, you may not want to use the incline, however.

STAIRCLIMBERS:

In my opinion, stairclimbing machines, found in most gyms, are one of the most effective pieces of aerobic equipment for reducing bodyfat and conditioning the heart. Stairclimbers are very efficient fat burners because they involve the large muscle groups in the legs, buttocks, and back.

The more that these larger muscles are incorporated, the greater your overall bodyfat reducing potential. Stairclimbing isolates the muscles of the thighs and buttocks, and is safer than running or jogging because there is less impact on the joints.

Personally, I have found that I obtain the quickest results when I dedicate myself to three back-to-back twenty minute sessions on the Stairmaster, taking stretching and water breaks between each round. For me, no other aerobic exercise works better for firming up the problem areas of the hips, thighs, and buttocks.

In all honesty, it took some time to comfortably build up to that level and I wouldn't recommend it for everyone. There are days when I skip the weights and the extended cardio sessions are all that I do because I feel that I have obtained a sufficient amount of exercise for that particular day.

Many people initially find stairclimbers to be difficult and sometimes give up on the equipment after using them only once or twice. You may be able to exercise longer than you realize on the stairclimbers, however, by beginning slowly (perhaps just five to ten minutes) and gradually increasing your time and resistance to safely work your way through the initial discomfort zone.

With practice, you will soon reach a comfortable pace and length of time where you are raising metabolism and burning off bodyfat. Do not cheat yourself by supporting your weight on the handrails. Use the handrails for balance if you must, but ideally you should lightly swing your arms to involve more muscle groups and increase cardiovascular strength.

Always maintain proper posture. Avoid leaning forward, since leaning puts unnecessary strain on the lower back. To avoid the tingling of the foot sometimes associated with stairclimbers, push through your heel on your down step while keeping your foot flat. For maximum benefit, flex your calves on the way up, as you rise to climb each step.

The three pieces of exercise equipment described above are just a few of the most popular ways of integrating aerobic exercise into your daily lifestyle. Fortunately, in today's world, there are a multitude of exercise options to choose from, and there is no excuse for allowing yourself to become stuck in an exercise rut.

The gym is certainly not the only place that you can obtain a good, heart-pumping workout. If you have tried health clubs and have found that they are simply not for you, then take a long walk or bike ride. If possible, choose a place with pleasant scenery, that helps connect you with the healing energy of nature.

Depending on the weather and your location, there are plenty of exciting exercise alternatives to chose from, such as mountain biking, running, hiking, snowboarding, downhill and cross country skiing, swimming, surfing, climbing, tennis, baseball, soccer, basketball, water aerobics, tai chi, or yoga.

Buy or rent a pair of inline skates and call a friend to join you for an invigorating spin around the neighborhood. Go for an exhilarating mountain bike ride or play basketball with your buddies. Instead of watching sports on television, get out there and do something while you still can!

Since balance is a crucial component of your Pura Vida lifestyle, it is important to combine the *yin* of softer, relaxing activities such as meditative swimming or gentle walking, with the *yang* of more forceful exercises, such as weight training or racquetball. Variety is the spice of life, and is as important in your exercise program as it is in your diet.

Engaging in several different types of sports, exercises and activities on a regular basis, sometimes defined as cross training, can add excitement and variety to your exercise program, which will keep you from becoming bored and possibly quitting. Mixing your exercise routine up with cross training not only keeps the exercise portion of your Pura Vida lifestyle from becoming too predictable, but participating in different activities, exercises, and sports works different muscle groups and varies the amount of aerobic and anaerobic exercise that you obtain.

Think back to when you were a child, always moving, running, and playing. Most likely, you did not have to make a conscious effort to stay active. It simply came natural to you to want to have fun and move your body. No matter what age you are, you probably still have a little kid spark left in you that has not been smothered by our work oriented culture.

In general, our society has a tendency to measure life mainly in terms of how much you produce or what material possessions you own and puts very little value on the quality of your life experiences. You should not feel guilty about spending time enjoying the precious gift of pure life or tending to your health and well-being.

Sometimes, your everyday responsibilities and worries may seem so overwhelming that you cannot imagine taking the time to go for a bike ride with the kids or going for a long, meditative walk. When you do not make the time to take care of your body and nourish your soul, however, you are shortchanging yourself in the long run.

Ironically, you will be missing out on some of the very things that can make you stand out from the crowd, and give you a competitive edge in today's prove yourself world. Consistent energy, endurance, and an attractive, fitter body are just a few of the practical benefits you will gain by making regular exercise a high priority in your new Pura Vida lifestyle.

Have you ever found yourself admiring a beautiful celebrity like Julia Roberts or studied a graceful athlete such as Tiger Woods performing at the peak of his game and silently wondered if perhaps they are privy to some health and fitness secrets that we mere mortals will never know about? I certainly have.

Perhaps the answer to the previous question has something to do with the fact that those charmed few in the elite ranks of the entertainment and sports industry truly understand the importance of maintaining a strong, healthy, well tuned body in today's world.

In our highly competitive, youth oriented society, the entire career of a world class or professional athlete rides on the state of his or her physical condition at any given moment. It is imperative that their bodies operate at 100 percent of their peak potential in order to stay at the top of their often short lived careers.

Also, as those who regularly bask in the glow of the Hollywood limelight have recently discovered, if you don't take care of your body and keep it looking great, you are very likely to lose roles that end up going to younger, more physically fit actors and actresses.

In addition, demanding shooting schedules and expensive filming deadlines do not allow much room for delays caused by stiff necks, headaches, and low back pain, so pain prevention is crucial for today's entertainers and athletes alike. Perhaps that is part of the reason that celebrities and athletes have so wholeheartedly embraced Holistic health care systems.

On a deeper, more spiritual level, you will also be creating memories that will last a lifetime when you venture out into the great outdoors, exercising your physical body, quieting your busy mind, and connecting with your pure life spirit. One of my most treasured memories is of an eventful day that Len and I spent with lifelong friends three days before our wedding. We all began the day with a stimulating and challenging, four hour mountain bike ride through the rugged trails of the New River Gorge, a wild and scenic wilderness area in the lush mountains of West Virginia.

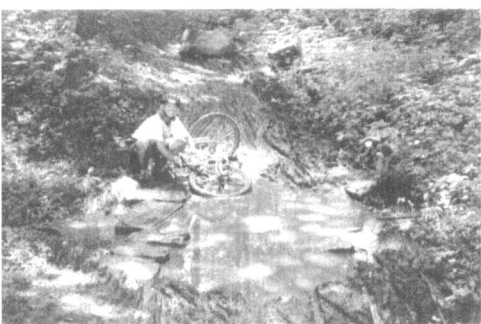

At the end of this gloriously muddy ride, we donned life jackets and hopped into a raft, paddling for the rest of the day through some of the most exciting rapids in the country, on one of the oldest rivers in the world. We laughed, engaged in juvenile water battles, knocked each other off the raft, shrieked in genuine fear, jumped off cliffs, and paddled until our arms felt like wet noodles, ending the day cold and exhausted but profoundly content.

During the course of our lives, we have been fortunate to have experienced some of the so-called finer things in life; traveling across the country at least thirty times in a private jet, sampling some of the world's best restaurants, and staying in some of the country's best hotels. Yet, those memories somehow pale in comparison to the sometimes challenging, fun filled Pura Vida adventures that we have experienced in the great outdoors.

At times like these, there is a feeling that can only be described as a heightened state of awareness, where we have felt a deep, powerful connection to the earth and to our own inner energy. Perhaps you too have experienced this phenomenon, and possibly felt as if time were slowing down or standing still, or noticed that colors are brighter or that your environment appeared more vivid and clear.

Fortunately, these moments do not have to take place in amazing wilderness areas or exotic locales. They can be experienced right now in the privacy of your own backyard or in a public park amongst hundreds of other people.

I often feel an indescribable sense of well being while simply taking a long walk on the beach near my home. At times, it almost seems that there is a palpable contented energy emanating from other beachgoers, and I wonder if it might have something to do with the fact that everyone is there because they truly want to be there. Many of them are tourists and have waited long periods of time for the opportunity to put their feet in the sand and read a good book or try their hand at windsurfing or fishing in the ocean.

You can't help but smile when you hear the laughter of children playing in the surf with uninhibited joy, perhaps for the very first time. It's only natural to feel a connection to the weathered, shyly grinning shell seekers because they radiate a sense of contentment and peaceful calm. No matter what kind of mood I am in when I start walking, I am always in a better mood when I finish.

Hopefully you are now incorporating what you learned from the tenth stepping stone by spending quality time in Nature, connecting with your life force, and breathing deeply. Build on these experiences and create even more memorable adventures by spending time outdoors exercising, moving your body, and engaging in sports and recreational activities.

There is only one way to create memories of quality time spent enjoying life to the fullest while basking in the magnificence of nature. These experiences do not usually come to you. You have to go out and make them happen.

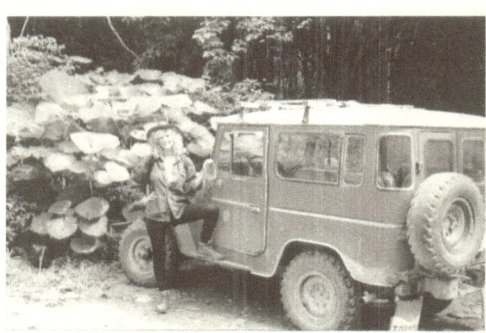

You, and only you, have the power to choose to explore your world and be open to new opportunities to stretch and exercise your mental, physical, and spiritual muscles.

Walking For Life

The human body is made to walk. All of the joints in your body, including your sacroiliac joints and the intricate joints of the vertebral column, work best when they are regularly taken through their normal ranges of motion during exercise and physical activity. Stiffening of the joints is often a result of insufficient movement, sometimes called the use it or lose it principle. Since your body was specifically designed to stride along in an upright position, walking is the most natural exercise there is.

A regular program of distance walking has also been proven to strengthen the cardiovascular system by lowering blood pressure and cholesterol. Reduced stress, increased muscle strength, improved digestion, and strengthened bones are just a few of the positive effects of consistently including walking in your daily lifestyle.

The beauty of walking is that all you really need is a proper pair of shoes. You can walk practically anywhere, at any time, and it can fit into most schedules. Since walking is a low impact, aerobic exercise, the risk of injury is minimal.

People are often surprised to learn that walking is one of the best exercises for strengthening the muscles of the back. Strong back muscles create stability in the spinal column and help keep the vertebrae in proper alignment. Walking also gives all of the muscles of the lower body—including the quadriceps, hamstrings, calves, and glutes—a good workout. By engaging in power walking, using light hand weights, you will involve more muscle groups, which increases resistance and muscle building potential.

How far and how fast should you walk? It depends on your goals, overall health, and physical strength. Start out slowly, using the first stepping stone as a touchstone, taking the time to listen to your body's innate intelligence. Gradually increase the distance that you feel comfortable walking briskly.

The faster you walk, the more positive benefits you will gain. If you are walking for overall health reasons, a general guideline is at least thirty minutes, three to five times a week. For people who are extremely overweight or new to exercise, walking is an ideal choice.

If your specific goal is to lose bodyfat, gradually increase your speed and work your way up to forty-five to sixty minutes, five or six days a week. If you are walking mainly for cardiovascular benefits, stride briskly enough to breathe hard, yet be able to hold a conversation for at least thirty to forty-five minutes.

Be aware of your form the next time you take a walk. Ask yourself the following questions. Is my head held high? Are my shoulders back? Is my stomach in? Am I taking long, fluid strides? Am I breathing deeply from my stomach?

Be sure not to hyperextend, or lock your knees, as you walk. Practice swinging your arms from the shoulders and elbows, which increases cardiovascular benefits and flexibility, and gives your upper body more of a workout.

Walking outdoors in fresh air, close to nature, gives you the added benefit of healthier lungs and a healthier mind. One of our favorite forms of exercise is hiking. Besides being a muscular and cardiovascular workout, there are the added benefits of a sense of exploration and adventure, and being in touch with the pure energy of nature. We have experienced some of our most memorable real moments while hiking in the mountains on crisp, magical fall days and fresh spring mornings.

Perhaps you also have some pleasant memories of walking down a sandy beach with the sun caressing your shoulders or striding happily along a sun-dappled, wooded trail. During those moments you may have been so in tune with your body that you thought, "This feels so good, I should do it more often." If you are feeling a little depressed or lethargic, put one foot in front of the other, get outside and start walking. There is an exciting world out there, just waiting to be discovered.

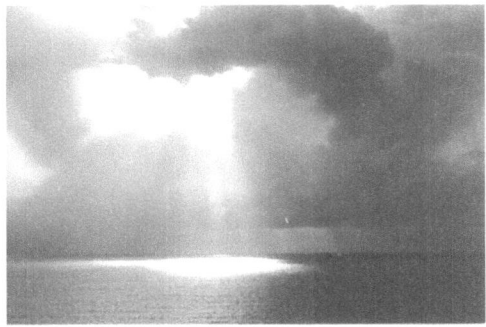

Muscle Anatomy

More than four hundred muscles help keep your body firm and strong. Fortunately, the stronger your muscles are, the more they help protect and reinforce the joints they support. Muscles are also necessary for controlling movement in the human body. The muscle that you can see directly under the skin is a specific type of tissue called striated or skeletal muscle. The contraction of striated muscle causes the skeleton to operate by using an amazing system of leverage.

It is important to be familiar with the muscles and their actions as you are performing every movement of any exercise. To help you better understand muscle anatomy, I have provided the following highlights. Hopefully, you will find muscle anatomy increasingly interesting as you become more aware of using specific muscles in your daily activities.

I have found that it can be quite thrilling for someone who has never given the subject much thought to discover that certain fibers of each muscle are responsible for specific actions or to watch a muscle contract and relax as you work it, fully aware of its name and function.

This was one of the factors that encouraged me many years ago to obtain a personal trainer's license in addition to my professional Chiropractic degree. At the time, the word trainer was only used in reference to sports training and not part of the popular lexicon as it is today. I simply had a passion for wanting to learn everything that there is to know about muscle anatomy and physiology. Of course, I'll never know or remember it all but I have certainly enjoyed the learning process and sharing it with others.

Being familiar with muscle anatomy will naturally make your strength training exercises more efficient and focused. Applying knowledge from both areas (muscle anatomy and strength training) often brings it all together for some people. For example, realizing that one of the functions of the biceps muscle is supination (turning the palm upward) and applying this knowledge while doing biceps curls, results in a more efficient, effective workout of that particular muscle.

I encourage you to use this section mainly as a reference guide. Do not worry about memorizing the exact names, locations, or functions of the muscles listed below. Instead simply read over this section and then refer to it as often as you wish until you are familiar with the major muscles and their actions.

SHOULDERS:

The *Deltoid* is the large triangular muscle of the shoulder that forms the visible rounded flesh of the outer part of your upper arm. The deltoid muscle forms a shape resembling an inverted triangle in people with highly defined musculature. It passes up and over your shoulder joint. The deltoid muscle is made up of three portions: the *Anterior* (front) *Deltoid*, the *Medial* (middle) *Deltoid*, and the *Posterior* (rear) *Deltoid*.

The action of the deltoid muscle is to raise your arm upward. The anterior fibers raise your arm to the front. The medial fibers raise your arm straight out to the side, and the posterior fibers lift your arm to the rear.

The group of muscles responsible for stabilizing the shoulder joint is commonly called the rotator cuff. These are the shoulder muscles often injured in sports, for example, by throwing a baseball or serving a tennis ball. The rotator cuff consists of four small muscles: the *Supraspinatus, Infraspinatus, Teres Minor,* and *Subscapularis* muscles, sometimes called the SITS muscles.

BACK:

The *Trapezius,* commonly called the *traps,* is a broad, flat, diamond shaped muscle that covers the upper and back part of your neck and shoulder region. Your trapezius muscle runs from the base of the skull to the mid-portion of the back. The upper trapezius is perhaps the most common spot for muscular tension and is also the muscle that makes some bodybuilders look like they have no neck due to over development of the muscle.

The upper, highly visible section of your traps elevates the shoulders, as in shrugging your shoulders. The middle section draws your shoulder blades together, and the lower section lowers your shoulder blade.

The *Rhomboid Major and Minor*, commonly called the *rhomboids*, lie in the upper back under the traps. Acting together with the middle and lower fibers of the traps, the rhomboids pull your shoulder blades back toward the spine. Considering their location and actions, it is easy to see why strong rhomboids and traps are essential for good posture.

The *Latissimus Dorsi,* also known as the *lats*, are the largest muscles of the upper body, and extend from under the shoulders down to the small of your back on both sides. The lats form the upper portion of the V-shape in a well-developed back. The basic function of the lats is to pull your shoulders downward and to the rear, as in rowing a boat or swimming. Competitive swimmers usually have nice, highly developed lats.

The *Quadratus Lumborum* is a very large, deep muscle of the lower back that helps you bend forward at the waist. It has no cute nickname but is extremely important for spinal stability.

The *Erector Spinae* consists of several muscles that form a long, thick muscle mass running from the top of your neck to the small of your back. These muscles are vital for spinal column stability and help you to stand in an erect posture, bend, and twist.

CHEST:

The chest is covered mainly by the *Pectoralis Major,* a thick, fan shaped muscle divided into upper and lower parts. The Pectoralis major has the action of drawing your arms forward, and bringing them across the front of your chest in a hugging type motion. The *Pec Major,* as it is often referred to, is also used to raise, lower and rotate the arms.

The action of the smaller *Pectoralis Minor* (a.k.a. *Pec Minor*) is to draw your shoulder blade downward and inward, and to bring your arm down and across your chest. Together, the pectoralis major and pectoralis minor, often referred to simply as the *pecs* make up the biggest part of your chest.

ARMS:

Your arm, which includes the upper arm below the shoulder, and also the forearm, consists mainly of the *Biceps brachii* (*biceps*), the *Triceps brachii* (*triceps*), and the forearm muscles. Named for its two heads (the long and the short head), the biceps muscle (nicknamed *bi's*) is located on the front of your upper arm and runs from your shoulder to your elbow. The biceps has the function of turning your palm upward (supination), and flexing your elbow joint.

The triceps muscle is found in the back of your upper arm and is made up of three teardrop shaped heads (the long, lateral, and medial heads). The triceps muscle is the main extensor of your elbow joint, and is used in actions that involve extending or straightening your arm.

To help you distinguish between the bi's and tri's, just remember that the biceps are the Popeye muscles in the front of the arms, which flex the elbow joints. The triceps are in the often jiggly area in the back of the arms. You may know the area as the one that keeps waving goodbye even after you have quit. The tris have just the opposite action (extending the elbow joint) of the bis (flexing the elbow joint).

If you have trouble differentiating flexion and extension, again think of the Popeye biceps muscle of the arm. To flex your biceps, you are bringing the two bones closer together, or decreasing the angle. Extension is simply the opposite of flexion. During extension, you are increasing the angle between the two bones. Extension often means a straightening out of the joint.

Your forearms are composed of several small muscles, including the *Brachioradialis,* which is located on the outer part of your forearm. The main action of the brachioradialis muscle is to help your biceps bend the forearm at the elbow joint. The brachioradialis (no catchy nickname that I know of) is often involved in tennis elbow type injuries.

ABDOMINALS:

Your *abs* (short for abdominal muscles) are made up of several different muscles. The *Rectus Abdominus* is a long, flat muscle that extends vertically the entire length of your abdomen, creating the washboard look (if you are working these muscles extremely hard or simply genetically blessed). The primary action of this muscle is to flex the spine, allowing you to bend forward at the waist.

The action of the upper portion of this muscle is to draw your breastbone towards your pelvis. The lower portion of the rectus abdominus helps draw your hips toward your ribs. Keep these actions in mind while you are doing crunches.

The *Transversus Abdominus* is a deeper muscle that runs horizontally beneath your rectus abdominus. It assists in breathing and helps to hold the organs in place.

The *Serratus Anterior* is the large muscle that looks like little serrated fingers curving along the outer portion of the ribcage in a well-developed person. You use this muscle when you reach out or push forward with your arms.

The *Internal and External Oblique* muscles are used when you twist your torso and bend your spine, such as in doing crunches with a twist. The external oblique is the larger of these muscles, which are commonly referred to as the *obliques.* The external oblique runs along the side and partly on the front of your torso. This muscle is usually concealed by bodyfat or love handles (also known as *lovis handelus*). Just kidding!

BUTTOCKS:

The powerful *Gluteus Maximus* is the strongest muscle in your body, but for many of us it is the most underdeveloped. This underdevelopment or sagginess is often the result of years of sitting and inactivity. The gluteus maximus covers a large part of your buttocks and is used when you extend your thigh. This muscle is used for walking, running, climbing, and rising from a seated position.

The *Gluteus Medius* is partly covered by the gluteus maximus. The function of this muscle is to move your thigh away from your body and to rotate your leg inward. Located under the gluteus medius, lies the tiny *Gluteus Minimus*, a small buttocks muscle that has the same action as the gluteus medius.

The gluteus maximus, medius, and minimus are often referred to simply as the *glutes*, and are the muscles to specifically work on in order to strengthen, lift, and tighten the buttocks (also known as the buns, bum, butt, or fanny). Just checking to make sure that you are paying attention!

LEGS:

Your powerful legs consist mainly of three basic muscle groups: the quadriceps in the front of the thigh, the hamstrings in the back of the thigh, and the muscles of the calves. The *Quadriceps* (also known as the *quads*) is composed of the four muscles in the front and sides of the upper leg: the *Rectus Femoris*, and the three vastus muscles of the quads, specifically the *Vastus Lateralis, Vastus Medialis,* and *Vastus Intermedius.* The basic function of your quads is to extend or straighten your leg, as in kicking a ball. Strong quads help stabilize your knee joint.

Together, these four important muscles connect your pelvic bone and your upper leg bone, coming together to form the Patellar Tendon. This tendon crosses over the front of your knee and inserts into your kneecap (technically known as the Patella).

The patellar tendon is the tendon that the doctor hits with his (or her) hammer to elicit the knee jerk reflex. While we are on the subject of reflexes, here is an interesting tidbit of information about neural anatomy and physiology involving the patellar tendon that I have always found quite astounding.

If you have ever wondered why your leg kicks uncontrollably when hit at just the right angle at the patellar tendon, consider this. A reflex is your innately intelligent body's way of protecting itself in emergency situations, such as when you place your hand on a hot stove. When you are in danger of severing the tendon connecting your muscles to the bone at the knee joint (and also at other tendon insertion sites, such as the Achilles Tendon of the ankle joint), the reflex action takes over.

The reflex bypasses the normal, slower route of sending information up the spinal cord to the brain to be processed, then sending information back down the spinal cord, and out through the spinal nerves to whatever part of the body it wants to move quickly in order to avert physical harm.

Put simply, a reflex basically sends the information to the spinal cord and back out, without traveling up and down the cord as it normally does, and then being analytically processed by the brain, saving valuable time in survival situations.

Now, let us move around to the back of the upper leg. There are three hamstring muscles in the back of your thigh: the *Biceps Femoris*, and the two *Semi* muscles of the hamstrings, specifically *Semimembranosus, and Semitendinosus.*

To reiterate what you learned earlier, your quads consist of the rectus femoris muscle and the three vastus muscles. Your hamstrings consist of the biceps femoris and the two semi muscles. The main function of the hamstring group of muscles is to flex your knee (curl your leg back). They also help to extend your thigh.

Having a nice set of hamstrings accentuates the leg and buttock area, creating a well-proportioned look. Strengthening and shaping the hamstring muscles rebuilds the structure underneath fat deposits on the back of the thigh. This firm muscle tissue makes fat deposits appear smoother and less obvious. More importantly, strong hamstring muscles also help stabilize and protect your lower back.

The two major muscles that form your calves are the *Gastrocnemius* (sometimes called the *gastrocs*) and the *Soleus,* which lies underneath the gastrocnemius. These muscles work together with a few others to flex your foot, or point your toe, and to push with your feet. Both calf muscles attach to your ankle by the achilles tendon. The deeper, wider soleus is used for endurance exercises, such as running. The more visible, rounded gastroc comes into play during activities such as jumping.

The *Tibialis Anterior,* located on the outer side of your leg along your shinbone, attaches to the bones of your ankle and foot. The primary function of this muscle is to move your foot upward. Stretching the tibialis anterior muscle can help prevent painful shin splints.

Last but not least, you have probably heard about the *abductor* and *adductor* muscles and machines, which can be a little confusing. The *Abductor* muscles are located on the outer portion of your upper legs, while the *Adductors* are located on your inner thigh.

I remember these actions like this: *ADD*uctors add or bring the legs closer to the middle of the body, as when you bring your legs together during activities such as horseback riding. Conversely, abductor muscles help move your leg away from the midline of your body.

Since a woman's body is naturally designed to store bodyfat in the inner and outer thigh, they can benefit tremendously by strengthening the adductor and abductor muscles, which make fatty deposits in these areas appear less noticeable.

Hopefully, the above information has helped you become more familiar with the location and actions of most of the major muscles and muscle groups of your body. This knowledge will make it easier to see which particular exercise or combination of exercises you need to perform in order to target specific muscles or muscle groups. For instance, knowing that the gluteus maximus is used for rising from a seated position, or that the deltoid raises the arm, helps you to understand why certain exercises work specific muscles as well as specific areas of the body.

This knowledge can help you to effectively target your problem areas with precision and intensity. Use this powerful information to your advantage to add a deeper understanding and focus to your exercise program and in your everyday healthy, active lifestyle.

Strength Training With Weights

We have all encountered resistance along our own unique paths through life that eventually helped form our character and made us stronger individuals, who are much better equipped to handle the next unexpected challenge that comes our way. The same is true of building muscles with weights or strength training.

Not only can you make your physical body stronger by applying resistance to your muscles with the use of machines or free weights, but you can also dramatically change your outward appearance and increase your level of self confidence.

Like any other living thing, your body naturally adapts to a certain amount of stress placed on it. If you perform hard labor using your hands, the skin will eventually harden and gradually develop calloused areas. Likewise, when you place a considerable amount of resistance on your muscles through the use of strength training with free weights or machines, your body naturally makes the muscles stronger in order to be ready for the next time they are needed.

The process of building muscle tissue is quite fascinating and somewhat complicated. Basically, however, what happens is this: during a process called catabolism, your muscle tissue is naturally broken down as it is placed under a certain amount of stress or resistance, such as lifting a heavy weight. As the tissue rebuilds and repairs itself during a process called anabolism, it builds back a little bit stronger, in order to be ready for the next overload.

If you are between the ages of thirty and thirty-five, you may find it interesting (and also quite unfair) to know that muscle mass tends to begin slowly decreasing at this age. Around age fifty-five, muscle mass tends to decrease even more rapidly. These facts are especially relevant if you are trying to lose bodyfat, since muscle is the body's most metabolically active tissue. Also, strong muscles reinforce and stabilize joints, helping to prevent injury, stiffness, and pain. These are just a few of the reasons why the next stepping stone on your journey involves strength or weight training.

Although the original Pura Vida Path builders may not have had access to modern weight training equipment, the principles of strength training that they incorporated naturally in their active daily lives remains the same. I encourage you to fully utilize the power of the next stepping stone, which helps form the sturdy, multi-tiered ledge made up of the four integrally related exercise stepping stones.

Stepping stone # 15: *Strengthen the muscles and bones of your body with the use of resistance or weights on a regular basis.*

The results that you will obtain while strength training are usually in line with the law of Pure Energy balance. In other words, you will get out of it what you put into it.

Weight training, sometimes known as dynamic or isotonic training, includes two different components of muscle contraction: *concentric* and *eccentric* contractions. A good example of the concentric component of a muscle contraction is the curling action of a dumbbell curl. During this concentric portion of the muscle contraction, the biceps muscle shortens as it contracts to move the weight while you raise the dumbbell upward.

The eccentric component of muscle contraction, on the other hand, involves the lengthening of a muscle. For example, the lowering action of a dumbbell curl, during which the arm is slowly straightened from a bent position, is considered as the eccentric component of the dumbbell curl exercise.

The eccentric component is also known as negative contraction, and is commonly referred to as doing negatives in gym settings. To increase the size of a particular muscle, it helps to focus your energy on the eccentric type of contraction during each repetition. This is a simple, effective tip that is often overlooked by many people who are quickly rushing through their weight training exercises, and wondering why their muscles are not growing larger.

The term isometrics refers to a muscle contraction in which the muscle length is unchanged. In contrast to the concentric and eccentric contractions that occur in dynamic activities such as weight training, an isometric contraction occurs in activities involving squeezing and holding the muscles. For example, pushing against a doorframe or other immovable object without moving the joints of your arm would involve an isometric contraction.

Since each of us has a unique body structure, health history, and distinctly different goals, I feel that it is unwise for any two individuals to follow the exact same strength training program. Like every other aspect of your Pura Vida Lifestyle, you must seek and find the specific path that is uniquely right for you at this particular time in your life. As you evolve and change, so will your activity level, exercise program, and health related goals.

Every muscle in your body performs a specific action or actions. For example, one of the actions of your bicep muscle is to bend the arm by bringing the forearm toward the arm, as in pulling weeds or carrying heavy objects. When you are strength training with weights, you are actually simulating the normal, every day action of specific muscles or muscle groups.

The most efficient way to strengthen specific areas of your body with weights, therefore, is to learn the action of the muscle or muscles in that particular area and find a safe, efficient strength training exercise that duplicates that specific action.

Over the years, I have found one simple rule to be of utmost importance when working out with weights. When you focus your energy on using proper, safe form instead of focusing on the amount of weight that you are using, you will see much more consistent, positive results while strength training. It is much more effective and safe to practice correct form as described in the following chapters, and to carry the movement through its full range of motion than it is to keep adding plates on the stack.

In strength training terms, a repetition (or rep) is simply the number of times that you perform a particular exercise. The amount of *repetitions* (or *reps*) that you do is a key factor in determining how your body will be shaped during weight training. To achieve overall toning and definition, it is recommended that you use less weight and perform a higher number of repetitions. To gain bulk or size you should use heavier weight and do fewer reps. you should raise or lower the amount of weight that you use to conform to the desired number of repetitions—not the other way around.

If you are attempting to create or maintain muscle tone or definition, I recommend using a weight that you feel comfortable lifting for twelve to fifteen repetitions. The last two or three reps of that set (in this example, the set is a group of twelve or fifteen reps) should require extra effort.

If your goal is to add bulk or size to your muscles, I recommend using a weight that you are comfortable lifting for six to eight repetitions. The last one or two reps of the set should require quite a bit of extra effort. For example, if your goal is to increase the size of your biceps muscle, you could perform eight bicep curls in a row, or eight repetitions. Each time you do eight curls in a row, this is considered a set.

The speed at which you perform your repetitions is crucial. To avoid rushing through your workout, practice what you have learned from the third Stepping stone by finding your calm center, and taking the time to count slowly and breathe deeply from your stomach. In some instances, it helps to briefly close your eyes in order to focus on connecting with your inner energy. By unleashing your powers of concentration, and making every rep count, you will also be strengthening your mental muscles.

A good guideline for performing repetitions of most strength training exercises is using a two to one ratio. Following the same bicep curl example as above, you would slowly count to four while lowering the arm during the negative (eccentric) part of the exercise. When the negative is controlled and performed slowly, there is less assistance from gravity and more muscle-building resistance.

Then, while bending the arm and curling the biceps in the concentric portion of this exercise, you would slowly count to two seconds, while lifting the dumbbell and squeezing the biceps muscle, taking half as much time to raise the weight as you did to lower it.

People who are in hurry and rushing through their workouts often use the reverse of this two to one ratio. For instance, they would take more time for the curl than for the lowering action, which actually reduces the amount of muscle building potential by giving in to gravity's assistance on the way down.

Len and I have found that using a combination of free weights and machines works best for us. Free weights include dumbbells and round plates that are stacked equally on both sides of short or long bars, which are either straight or curled.

Some weight training machines also utilize free weight in the form of round plates. Many strength training machines utilize a large stack of rectangular plates, with the weight determined by placing an adjustable metal pin in the slot next to the poundage of weight that you desire for that particular exercise.

Regardless of the type of equipment that you are using, you should try to focus on working both sides of your body equally and evenly. You should be aware that a long straight bar, for example, and certain machines that work both sides of the body at the same time, can allow the strong side to overcompensate for the weaker side.

This inequality of resistance can eventually lead to an imbalance in the structural foundation of your body. A muscular imbalance of this type can be particularly detrimental when it involves the muscles surrounding and supporting the spinal column.

Once you become familiar with muscle anatomy, you are able to visualize the specific muscle contracting and relaxing with each movement. This helps you to target that particular muscle much more effectively than simply going through the motions.

In addition, touching the muscle you are working helps to establish a unique neural pathway linking the brain to that specific muscle. Every time you repeat this process, the link between your amazing brain and that particular muscle is reinforced via the intricate, winding paths of the nervous system.

Of course, it is not always convenient or necessary to touch every muscle that you are exercising. You may simply want to lightly hold your hands on your thighs as you do leg extensions, or gently squeeze your bicep muscle between sets of bicep curls to bring added focus to the muscle or muscle group involved.

No matter what type of weight training you perform to strengthen your muscles, it is very important that you also incorporate aerobic activity into your healthy Pura Vida Lifestyle. This combination not only maximizes excess body fat loss, but also keeps the inside of your body as healthy as the outside.

Despite what countless videos may tell you, there is no such thing as spot reducing. When fat is metabolized or burned, it is burned from all over the body. Fat is not reduced selectively in only the exercised areas, but rather from the total bodyfat reserves.

Spot strengthening, on the other hand, is possible. You can target certain areas to add more muscle, but not specifically to lose excess body fat. As you already know, the more lean muscle you have, the more efficiently fat is burned throughout your entire body.

Combining regular cardiovascular exercise with a consistent strength training program can be accomplished in a number of different ways, depending on your current fitness level, lifestyle, and personal goals.

Some fitness experts recommend always performing your aerobic exercise before strength training and others feel strongly that you should do your cardio only after your weights. In my opinion, what matters most is that you find some time in your busy life to give your heart and lungs a healthy workout. Whether that time is before or after your strength training workout is not as important as making sure that regular aerobic exercise and physical activity are an integral part of your daily lifestyle.

In reference to strength training with weights, if your goal is overall toning or you are limited to the amount of days that you can work out, you may find that a program in which you work the whole body each session works best for you.

One disadvantage to working all body parts during every workout is that there is less focus on each individual muscle group or body part. Another disadvantage is that you may not allow sufficient recovery time for the muscles to repair themselves, which is generally around forty-eight hours for an intense workout. Since the process of repairing and rebuilding of muscle fibers is what makes them grow, it is important to incorporate a healthy resting period for specific muscle groups.

Personally, Len and I have found that the most effective program is to work different body parts in each session. Like most people, the number of days per week that we work out with weights varies. As we have all experienced, it is often challenging to stay on an exact schedule in the real world. Unexpected events, delays, travel, family and work commitments, and a multitude of other reasons can prevent the best of intentions from being carried out.

Ideally, we have found that we look and feel our best when we do some type of resistance training four or five days a week. The intensity and duration of our workouts varies, with a few light days mixed in with more aggressive days, and is affected by the amount of cross training that we do in addition to strength training.

Below is an example of one of our weight training schedules based on a four day cycle. Notice that I use day numbers, such as day 1, day 2, etc. rather than days of the week because I have found that trying to always work chest on Mondays or legs on Wednesdays can be confusing and frustrating. If you have to miss a day, such as missing chest day on Monday, it throws off your entire schedule.

With a four-day cycle, if you must miss a day, you simply pick up on the next day of your routine and carry on. For example, regardless of what day of the week it is, on day 1 of a new four day cycle, you could put your full attention toward working out your chest and back.

On day 2, you might want to concentrate on triceps and biceps. Day 3 could be shoulder and calf day. Then, on day 4, work quads and hamstrings exclusively. After day 4, you could start all over with day 1 again, working chest and back. This type of cycle also gives the individual muscles sufficient time to rest between workouts.

If your goal is to have larger muscles, it is very important to add variety to your weight training program. You can achieve this goal by varying the amount of weight that you use and also varying the combination and types of exercises that you perform.

If you never change your routine, eventually, your muscles will adapt to whatever resistance is placed on them. Try to change your routine at least every six weeks or so, while mixing the order of the individual exercises daily.

Instead of working the abdominal muscles on separate days, we often work them moderately several days in a row. In our experience, abs and calves do not require as much rest as other muscle groups. It is a good idea to work your abs last, since they are important stabilizing muscles. You may risk injury if they are fatigued from working your abdominal muscles early in your workout.

Warming up, which includes stretching, is crucial before any type of serious exercise. Stretching is especially important if you have been inactive all day before beginning weight training exercises. Your muscles are more susceptible to micro tears when they have not been sufficiently stretched and loosened up prior to placing the resistance of weights on the joints and supporting muscles.

Also, just as you make adjustments before driving a car, you should always take the time to make adjustments to each machine before using it. Adjusting equipment to conform to your specific needs will help to maintain proper form throughout the exercise and prevent injury.

Fortunately, weight training, when performed correctly, is an excellent way to improve posture. By strengthening the muscles of the back that are directly related to supporting the spinal column, and also by strengthening muscles such as the hamstrings and abdominals, which help support the pelvis, poor posture can be significantly improved with regular weight training exercises.

Maintaining proper posture at all times is also crucial in achieving optimal results and preventing injury. While weight lifting, it is important to maintain the slight natural curves of the spine, which help make it stronger and more resil-ient. You should always avoid excessive arching or rounding of the lower back and instead strive for a neutral position, maintaining the slight natural forward curve in the neck and the lower back. An excessively arched lower back can place undue stress on the spinal joints, discs, and nerves.

Even if you are just beginning a weight training program, invest in a weight belt. It may save you from a serious injury by helping to support and stabilize your lower back. A precaution you should keep in mind when wearing a weight belt is not to lift more than you normally would without it. In other words, do not let the belt provide you with a false sense of security.

Remember to use the same proper lifting form that you use in your weight training while loading and unloading plates on and off the rack. Use your legs and keep the plates close to your body. (For more information on proper lifting technique, please see chapter 36.)

Since building muscle is all about resistance, it is imperative to maintain steady, continuous tension on the muscles as you perform each repetition of strength training exercises. To keep resistance constant, you should avoid coming to a complete stop at the top of an exercise, since stopping at the top lessens resis-tance and allows the muscle too much time to rest.

For example, during the biceps curl, you should not bring the forearm as far as it will bend in order to touch the upper arm and allow it to rest at the top of the curl. Instead you should stop short of that point and immediately begin the negative, downward portion of the exercise in a steady, controlled manner.

You should also avoid completely straightening or locking out the elbows or knees, which allows the resistance on the involved muscles to slacken and puts pressure directly on the joints. For example, during a bench press in which you are lying flat on a bench while holding dumbbells and raising both arms upward toward the ceiling, many people often completely straighten or lock out their elbows at the top of this exercise and rest for a brief moment.

In this locked position, the bones of the forearm and arm are lined up with one directly on top of the other and the joints are holding up the weight with little resistance on the muscles. Also, locking out the knees while performing most exercises puts undue stress and pressure on the delicate tissues of the lower back and can adversely affect the sciatic nerve, which exits from the lower portion of the spine and runs down the back of the leg.

Another important factor to keep in mind while weight training is to rely on muscle, not momentum, to move the weights. Do not cheat yourself by using a momentum-aided windup with every repetition. Instead, concentrate on using smooth, steady, controlled motions while lifting the weight without swinging your arms or legs past the proper range of motion for that particular exercise in an effort to gain speed and momentum.

By applying the information you learned from the third stepping stone concerning deep breathing, you can create a strong, direct link between your powerful mind and your sweaty physical body as you work out. Utilize the experience that you have gained thus far on your Pure Life journey to focus your energy on your breathing and visualize your body becoming stronger and healthier. Continually remind yourself to breathe deeply from your stomach as you are working out. Holding your breath while lifting a heavy object not only creates internal pressure, but it deprives your body of oxygen necessary to give you the extra power needed to make the lift.

If you are just beginning a weight training program, how quickly you will see results depends largely on how committed, consistent, and focused you are. Like every other aspect of your Pura Vida lifestyle, physical growth does not take place overnight.

Becoming physically stronger is a gradual ongoing process, which is affected either positively or negatively by all of the other integrally related components of your daily lifestyle. What matters most is that you treat your body with respect and concentrate on building balanced and lasting strength of your body, mind, and spirit.

Weight Training Exercises That Work

Len and I have both enjoyed the benefits of strength training since our teenage years, with a combined total of over twenty-five years spent consistently working out. Like many people, we have gone through periods or phases when we were more serious about weight training than others, but neither of us has ever strayed very far from a gym. We actually met in a gym, as a result of a series of synchronistic events, but that is another story, perhaps another book.

Throughout the years, through research, experimentation, and practical application, I have found certain strengthening exercises to be more effective than others and would like to share this information with you. In this chapter, I have highlighted some of my favorite exercises and answered some of the questions that I have been asked most frequently over the years. If the details of the particular exercises are not of special interest to you at this time, please regard this section as you have previous reference sections, lightly reading over it and coming back to spend more time at your convenience.

If you are just beginning weight training and are unfamiliar with the different types of exercises and equipment, I urge you to do further research in addition to studying the information contained in this book.

Since there is an inherent risk of injury involved in strength training, you should take this activity seriously and learn everything you can about safety and proper form. Using the services of a certified personal trainer can help you overcome any fear you might have of lifting weights and also help prevent unnecessary injuries. A professional trainer can serve as a good source of encouragement, advice, and information.

I have always believed that a good trainer is a good teacher and that a true teacher is not necessarily the one with the most knowledge, but the one who shares that knowledge with others in a practical way. Be careful not to become too dependent on a trainer or anyone else for your motivation, however. The positive driving force in your strength training program should come from within.

If you are already experienced in weight training, I suggest that you read this chapter to make sure that you are performing the exercises correctly and to see if there are any new exercises that you are not familiar with. By consistently performing the powerful exercises in this chapter, you can not only transform your physical body, but strengthen your mind and increase your self-confidence as well.

In this chapter, you will find some basic information about a few, but certainly not all, of the weight training exercises that I have found to be effective over the years.

CHEST:

The *flat bench press,* (usually known simply as bench press) is very effective for working the pectoralis or pec major muscle, using either a straight bar or dumbbells. Alternating techniques, by using the bar on one chest day, and dumbbells on the next chest day will work the fibers of the pec muscles in slightly different ways, and result in a more effective chest workout.

The ever popular question, "How much can you bench press?" should never enter your mind as you perform this exercise. Instead, the question should be, "How well can you bench press?" Determine how much weight to use by applying the principles explained earlier, adjusting the amount of weight and number of reps to your desired fitness goals.

To perform this exercise properly, lie flat on a bench with your knees bent and feet flat on the floor. If you are more comfortable bending your knees and placing your feet flat on the bench, you may also do so. I have found the bent knee position to be less stressful on the lower back. Holding a weight that is comfortable for you, grip your barbell firmly. When using a straight bar or barbell, keep your wrists directly above the elbows at the starting position, with your forearm perpendicular to your arm. A grip that is too narrow or too wide will put unnecessary strain on the shoulder and elbow joints.

Lift with a slow, smooth, controlled motion, breathing out on the way up. It is important to keep the workload in the muscles, not the joints, so be careful not to lock your elbows completely at the top. Locking out the elbow (or knee) joints overstretches the ligaments and puts most of the weight bearing pressure directly on the bones of the joint. When the elbow or knee is slightly bent, it brings the muscles into play to help support the joint and increase muscle-building resistance.

Lower the bar to the point where it just barely touches your chest. Keep the bar moving throughout the entire set, pausing only if necessary. If you have to arch your back excessively when you are lifting, you are using too much weight. Take some weight off and concentrate on proper form. Your hips should remain on the bench during the entire exercise. The same rules apply when using dumbbells.

In addition to the flat bench you may also want to do some *incline bench* work for the upper chest. A 45° angle bench angle works the upper chest effectively. An angle higher than 45° works the muscles of the shoulders more than those of the upper chest.

BACK:

The lat pull down, often referred to as pull downs, is an excellent exercise for strengthening the latissimus dorsi or lats and other back muscles. The lats are the muscles that help give a well-developed torso its V or spike shape.

To perform the lat pull down, hook up a wide, straight bar to the overhead cable. Choose a comfortable weight and grab the bar with a wide grip. Sit on the lat pull down machine with your knees under the pad. Your back should be straight, yet maintain its normal, slight natural curve. Slowly pull the bar down toward your uplifted chest, just clearing your chin.

It is important to make sure that you set or stabilize your shoulders before pulling down on the bar. Concentrate on pulling by using the lats first and then the arms. Tighten your abdominal muscles as you pull down to help support your lower back. Being careful not to rest too long at the position with the bar barely touching your chest, slowly release the bar to its starting position.

Always breathe deeply and continuously and use a smooth, controlled motion on the way up and down. Be aware of keeping your shoulders set as the bar is at its highest point, because you could possibly overstretch your shoulder joints by allowing the bar to go too far upward.

As someone who has treated thousands of patients with neck pain, I often cringe when I see people at the gym pulling the bar behind their neck on this exercise. This puts unnecessary strain on the shoulders and the delicate spinal tissue of the neck region. I highly recommend keeping it safe by staying away from this position and pulling to the front instead.

The *Seated cable row,* (usually called seated rows in a gym setting) is another excellent back exercise. The rowing motion of this weight training exercise effectively targets the lats and rhomboid muscles, which are essential for good posture. Concentrate on using these muscles instead of pulling with your arms alone.

Sitting close to the floor on the pad of the seated row machine, connect the small bar with the close double grip. Keep your knees slightly bent and your back straight (with its slight natural curve) throughout the entire exercise.

Use a weight that feels a little light until you are familiar with the motion and proper technique of this exercise. Lean forward and grab the bar with both hands. As you pull the bar toward your stomach, it is very important to keep your elbows in and back straight. Pull with a slow, controlled motion, breathing out as you pull. Maintain proper posture and do not collapse your upper body.

Concentrate on squeezing your shoulder blades together and pushing your chest forward as you pull the bar in with your arms. Keep your arms close to your torso. The only joints moving during this exercise should be the shoulders and elbows, not the back.

Keep the resistance as steady as possible while releasing slowly and returning to the starting position for a brief rest before the next repetition. Remember to set your shoulders before pulling backward on the next rep. As you are performing this exercise, visualize the results: strong rhomboids and lats, and confident, healthy posture.

TRICEPS:

The triceps muscles in the back of the upper arms are fairly easy to firm with some concentrated effort. Since excess bodyfat is readily stored in the triceps region, especially in women, it is important to build a solid foundation of muscle mass in this often ignored area.

One of my favorite triceps exercises is the *triceps press down*, using an overhead cable. Attach a short straight bar (or the short V-shaped bar) to one side of the cable crossover machine. Maintain proper posture, keep your shoulders back, and move only your elbow joints during this exercise. Keeping your elbows close to your sides, slowly press the bar toward the floor, while breathing out and pulling downward. Focus your energy on keeping resistance on the triceps muscles at all times.

Squeeze the triceps muscles at the bottom of the exercise, being careful not to lock out the elbows. Return to the starting point in a smooth, controlled manner. Visualize your triceps muscles becoming more well-defined and strong as you perform this exercise.

The popular *triceps kickback* exercise, most often simply referred to as kick backs, effectively works the lateral and medial heads of the triceps muscle. To work your left triceps muscle with the kickback exercise, you would place your right knee and right hand on a flat bench while bending forward. Your spine should be as close to parallel with the floor as is comfortably possible.

Begin the kick back movement by holding a light dumbbell in your left hand, with the upper part of your left arm parallel to the floor and your left forearm at a 90° angle to your upper arm.

Then, kick your arm back by slowly straightening your forearm backward, so that it is parallel with the floor. Do not lock out the elbow joint at this point, but rather keep a steady resistance on the triceps muscle. Gently squeeze the triceps muscle at the top of this movement while keeping resistance on the muscle constant. Avoid cheating by not using a swinging momentum.

To lower the weight, keep your upper arm in close to your body, bend your elbow, and drop your forearm in a slow, controlled manner. Stop when your forearm is at a right angle with your upper arm.

BICEPS:

My favorite biceps exercise is probably the world's most famous weight lifting exercise, the *standing biceps dumbbell curl*, (or just plain curls). This is the exercise that I have been using frequently as an example throughout the weight training and exercise portions of this book.

Stationary shoulder placement is a must in any type of biceps work. Stand with your back straight, shoulders down and back, and knees slightly bent. Place a dumbbell in each hand at your side, palms facing your body.

Slowly curl the dumbbell (one at a time or both) upwards toward your shoulder. As you curl, twist your palms outward slightly, so that they face you at the top. Remember to breathe out as you pull up. Keep the resistance constant and do not rest at the top. Squeeze the biceps muscle at the top, but do not curl your arm as far as it will go. Maintain a steady torso and stable shoulders throughout this exercise. Return smoothly to the starting point, keeping the elbows close to the body.

A fact that few people are aware of is that one of the actions of the biceps muscle is supination of the forearm. In this case, supination means going from a position with the palm facing down to a position with the palm facing up. An easy way to remember this is the UP in the word sUPination. Pronation is simply the opposite of supination.

The *seated preacher curl* (or simply preacher curl) effectively works the biceps muscle and is another one of my favorites. To perform this exercise, load a curl bar (the bar shaped like a letter W) with your desired weight, and adjust the seat height so that your armpits are just above the top of the pad. If the seat is too high, you will pull with your shoulders instead of your biceps muscles.

Alternate grips, performing one set using the inside grip on the curl bar and the next set using the outside grip. Slowly pull the bar toward your chin, breathing out as you pull up and stopping before your forearm touches your arm. Focus on squeezing the biceps muscle at the top of this exercise.

Every time you squeeze or contract a muscle at the top of a weight training exercise, visualize that muscle becoming stronger and more defined. This visualization combined with the physical action of squeezing helps reinforce neural pathways to the brain and can actually result in more visible results in your strength training program.

Continue the seated preacher curl exercise by slowly lowering the curl bar. Remember your 2 to 1 ratio. Always avoid complete lock-out of the elbows. Remember to keep your shoulders firmly set as you perform this exercise. If you have difficulty doing this, you are probably using too much weight. Your elbow should be the main moving joint in this exercise.

SHOULDERS:

The most common shoulder exercises focus on the deltoid muscle, which is the muscle that makes up the largest visible mass of the shoulder area. Whether or not the front, middle, or rear portion of the deltoid is worked depends primarily on which direction the arm is raised: i.e., to the front, the side, or the rear.

To better understand this concept, lower your right arm to the side of your body and place your left hand on your right deltoid muscle. Without bending your elbow, raise your arm straight out in front of you. You will feel the front (anterior) portion of the deltoid tighten.

When you raise your arm straight up and away from your body, you will feel a tightening of the middle fibers of the delt. Reaching behind you contracts mainly the rear (posterior) fibers of the deltoid muscle.

The *seated military press* (or just military press) works mostly the middle (medial) deltoid muscle by pressing the weights upward directly over the shoulders. When raising any weight overhead, you should always be careful not to arch your back excessively.

Begin the seated military press by sitting on the edge of a flat bench with a dumbbell in each hand at your side. Then, bend your elbows and raise the dumbbells from the sides of your body to your shoulders, with your palms facing forward, and in line with your shoulders.

Slowly lift both dumbbells straight up over your shoulders toward the ceiling. Breathe out as you push up, exhaling on exertion. You should end in a position with your arms parallel to each other. Avoid locking your elbows or resting at the top of this exercise.

Remember to keep your back straight with its slight natural curve. In a controlled manner, slowly lower the weights back to the starting position, in line with the shoulders, and rest for a brief moment before performing the next rep.

Side lateral raises specifically strengthen the middle portion of the deltoid muscle. Begin this exercise by sitting on a flat bench with the dumbbells at your side. Use a relatively light weight. You may also stand while performing side laterals (as they are often called).

With a slight bend in your elbows, raise the dumbbells straight out from your sides until they are even with your shoulders and horizontal with the floor. Then, slowly lower the dumbbells. Maintain proper posture and keep your elbows slightly bent during the entire exercise.

Avoid the temptation to rely on momentum by quickly jerking your arms upward. Do not arch your back excessively, as you often see people doing in a gym setting. Concentrate on performing the exercise properly, keeping the motion slow and steady, with continuous resistance on the deltoid muscles.

To strengthen the important (but often ignored) rear delts, I recommend *rear lateral raises,* (not to be confused with side laterals). This position feels a little awkward at first but the exercise is very effective when performed correctly. Use a light weight since this is a small muscle. Begin by sitting on the far edge of a flat bench, with your body bent considerably at the waist. Start off in a position with the dumbbells hanging together in the space behind your knees.

Finish by raising the weights slowly outward and upward. Your torso should remain in the bent over position throughout the entire range of motion, keeping your elbows slightly bent throughout the entire exercise. Keep the resistance on the rear shoulder constant, and do not cheat by using momentum. Strict form is necessary here. If this exercise causes pain in your neck or back, do not continue doing it.

CALVES:

Have you ever noticed how overweight people often have large, well-developed calf muscles? This is because their calves support their total bodyweight on one leg with each step. Since the calf muscles are accustomed to weight bearing resistance in everyday walking, they must be worked harder than most muscles in order to increase their current size. To build mass in the calves, you may reduce the resting period between sets, and use heavier weights.

There are basically two types of exercises for the calves, each working a different muscle of the calf. They are the *seated calf raise* and the *standing calf raise.*

Since it crosses over the knee joint, the visible, large gastrocnemius muscle of the calf is worked primarily when the knee is not bent, because bending the knee relaxes the gastroc muscle. The standing calf raise works mostly the rounded *gastrocnemius* muscle and, to a lesser extent, the soleus muscle. The deeper *soleus* muscle of the calf is best worked when in a seated position, as with seated calf raises.

The seated calf raise can be done while sitting on a seated calf machine or while sitting on the edge of a bench with the balls of your feet on a block and weight resting on your knees. Adjust the amount of weight that you use on the seated calf machine to the reps necessary for your desired goal. In other words, if your goal is definition and toning, use a weight that you are comfortable lifting for a high number of reps. Conversely; you should use a heavier weight and lower number of reps if your goal is to add size to your calves.

To add resistance to a simple seated calf raise done without the aid of a machine, you can hold dumbbells on top of your quads, though this sometimes feels a little awkward. Firmly place the balls of your feet on the floor piece of the machine or on a block on the floor, and raise your heels until you feel a good squeeze in the calf. Be sure to use a full range of motion when performing this exercise.

I like to use a second squeeze at the top of this motion by raising the heels a little higher and contracting the soleus a second time. Be careful not to bounce or use jerky motions while performing seated calf raises. Lower your heels until you obtain a full downward stretch. High repetitions (up to twenty reps in some cases) are usually necessary to see visible definition with calf exercises.

To effectively work the large gastrocnemius or gastroc muscle (which forms the rounded outer appearance of the calf) I prefer the simple *Standing Calf Raise.* This exercise can be done by standing on a block in the gym or on a stair at home.

You can apply added resistance by holding a barbell on your shoulders, with or without added weight, or holding dumbbells in each hand in order to add size and bulk to the gastroc muscle. If your goal is simply increased definition, however, then usually the only weight necessary while doing calf raises on a stair or block is the weight of your body.

You can hold lightly onto the wall, a machine, or a pole in front of you for support. Raise your whole body straight upward in a vertical line, balancing your weight on the balls of your feet. Concentrate on squeezing the calf at the top of the motion, using the double squeeze if you like. Do not lock out the knees and use high reps (up to twenty-five for some people) for maximum results.

QUADRICEPS:

Leg extensions are probably the best exercise for isolating the quads, (the muscles in the front of the thigh) and for strengthening the muscles around the knee joint. This exercise is often recommended for rehabilitation of the knee, since the quad muscles support and stabilize the knee joint.

Sit in the leg extension machine with the front of your ankles under the pad, your weight loaded, your legs bent at a 90° angle to your thighs, and all machine adjustments made. Raise your leg up with a smooth, full range of motion, while avoiding locking out the knee.

Squeeze the quadriceps muscle for a few seconds at the top of the exercise, but do not allow the muscle time to rest before lowering the weight back down with a slow and controlled movement. Keep your buttocks firmly on the seat and maintain proper posture throughout the exercise.

Some machines allow the option of working one leg at a time, which I prefer, because it isolates the muscle in that particular leg and does not allow the stronger leg to overcompensate for the weaker one.

The *leg press* machine is a great exercise for strengthening the quadriceps and buttocks muscles. The explanation that follows is specifically for leg press machines which are designed to push the weight at an upward, inclined angle. Begin by loading your weight on the machine and positioning yourself in the equipment with your weight belt securely fastened and your feet raised above your torso.

A good angle for the backrest (if it is adjustable) is approximately 45°. To involve more of the gluteal (buttocks) muscles, place your feet high on the plate with your toes hanging slightly over. If you are not sure how much weight to use, always play it safe by starting out with a light weight. Position your feet shoulder width apart and slowly lower the weight downward, gradually bending your knees. Keep your knees parallel to each other throughout the exercise. If your knees bow inward, you are using too much weight.

Be careful not to overstretch the ligaments of the knee by going too far down. Stop when your lower legs are at a 90° angle to your thighs. Your thighs should not collapse onto your chest. I have seen people literally get stuck in that position and have to yell for help when using too much weight.

Without resting at the bottom, begin pressing upward, concentrating on maintaining proper posture. Keep your back pressed against the pad at all times. Remember not to lock out your knees at the top and always use slow, smooth, controlled motions.

Some leg press machines are designed to push the weights out at more of a horizontal angle while sitting upright. To perform this type of leg press, simply adjust the machine to your body while seated and place your feet on the footplate in front of you to activate the weights. Your knees will be bent toward your chest at this point.

Use a light weight to start. Push outward with your feet while supporting your back against the backrest. Do not lock out your knees while straightening your legs. Maintain resistance while slowly lowering legs back to starting, bent knee position.

Squats are very effective for working the large muscles of the upper leg and buttocks, but are potentially dangerous if too much weight or improper form is used. In my opinion, squats should only be done with proper form and a very light, comfortable weight in order to avoid injury to the knees and to the back muscles surrounding the fragile spinal nerves and discs.

If you have lower back problems, I believe that you should avoid doing squats and use a comparable exercise instead, such as the leg press machine, which involves less weight bearing pressure on the discs of the lower back.

Although I usually do not recommend that beginning exercisers start off a new strength training routine that includes squats, many people have been doing them for years and have no problems with the exercise, so, for them, here are a few things to keep in mind.

When doing squats, the important thing to remember throughout the entire range of motion is to keep the back straight with its slight natural curve. Make certain not to lean forward too far, and to keep your eyes straight ahead. To prevent soft tissue damage to the knee joint, never let the knees extend over the toe line.

Always start out slowly with light weight. Contrary to the position that you see many body builders use, you should keep your toes pointed straight ahead, rather than pointing them inward or outward at an angle. The knee is a hinge type joint and is not meant to be twisted while weight-bearing pressure is applied.

HAMSTRINGS:

Strengthening the hamstring and abdominal muscles not only improves your physical appearance but also helps stabilize the lower back and pelvis due to the attachment of the hamstring and abdominal muscles in these areas. The more stable the foundation of your spine is, the less chance you have of injury and subsequent back pain and inactivity.

The *prone hamstring curl* (or simply hamstring curls) is one of the best exercises for isolating the hamstring muscles. Lie face down (prone) on the bench of the hamstring machine, with your ankles under the ankle pads. Then, slowly pull your lower legs toward your buttocks.

I have found that it is less stressful on your neck if you do not support the weight of your head on your chin, arching your neck upward, but rather lower your head as far down as you comfortably can while performing this exercise.

Be careful not to let your rear end rise up from the bench as you are pulling your legs toward your buttocks. If it does, lower the weight and concentrate on pressing your hips downward into the bench. This stabilizes your pelvis and prevents cheating by involving the hip joints and muscles other than the hamstrings. Focus on moving only the knee joint. Your ankles should not hit your buttocks, but rather come about three-quarters of the way up.

Concentrate on the negative portion of this exercise, lowering the weight very slowly for maximum results. Be very careful not to use excessive weight since using heavy weight can strain the muscles of the lower back.

LUNGES:

(Note: Lunges were also previously described in Chapter 25 and the description that follows is the same. As I mentioned earlier, this exercise is also excellent for increasing core strength and balance.

Lunges target the muscles of the lower body, specifically the gluteal muscles and the quads. When done properly and consistently, lunges can help lift and tighten the buttocks and add attractive definition to the muscles of the thigh.

Although lunges can be done in a Smith machine or with a barbell, I usually recommend walking or traveling lunges because there is less direct compressive force on the spinal discs and because I prefer the continuous motion and resistance involved in this forward type of movement.

Lunges can be performed with your hands on your waist or by holding dumbbells at your sides. You can increase your resistance, which also increases muscle strength, by gradually using heavier dumbbells.

When you first begin doing walking lunges, feeling a little off balance is normal. You may want to start off with a light weight in each hand (three or five pounds) rather than no weight at all, because the weight will help you maintain your balance. Find a long stretch of floor area for walking lunges, rather than staying in one spot, lunging forward then back.

Stand tall with your feet shoulder width apart, and toes and eyes pointed straight ahead. It is very important to maintain proper posture and keep your abdominal muscles contracted for added support. Take a giant step forward with your right foot until your knee is directly in line over, or slightly behind your ankle joint.

Do not allow the knee to extend over the toe of your right foot. Your left knee should come close to, but not touch the floor. You should feel a gentle stretch in your left leg. Hold this position for a few seconds, and then take a slow, controlled step with your left leg. Continue lunging forward, pausing only when necessary for balance.

You should be traveling in a straight line, concentrating on technique and contracting the muscles of the legs and buttocks. When done properly, you will really feel this exercise working these major muscle groups.

If you do not have adequate floor space, you may prefer to do the stationary version of the lunge. Keep the same precautions in mind, not allowing the knee to extend over the foot, and maintaining proper posture.

Lunge forward with one leg at a time, holding weights if you prefer. The knee of the leg that is not moving forward (the back leg) should come close to, but not touch the floor at the bottom of this exercise.

Return to the starting position with both feet together and repeat the lunges with the same leg. Use high reps if your goal is definition and toning, and lower reps and more weight for increased muscle size. Repeat this process with the other leg, taking sufficient time to rest between sets.

ABDOMINALS:

Having a nice set of abs takes work, unless you are genetically blessed. Unfortunately, you cannot spot reduce fat in the abdominal area. When fat is burned, it is reduced throughout your body, not simply in selective areas. Doing sit-ups alone will not make your abs pop out, if they are covered by a thick layer of excess bodyfat.

Achieving a lean body composition with a healthy amount of muscle comes from the proper combination of good nutrition, aerobic exercise, and strength training. Abdominal exercises strengthen the ab muscles, but being lean will make the abdominal muscles appear more visible.

The most common and effective abdominal exercise is the *crunch*. I prefer doing crunches rather than full sit-ups because crunches isolate the rectus abdominus muscles with little wasted effort. Full sit-ups, on the other hand, rely on momentum and also work the hip and back flexing muscles, which take some of the muscle building resistance off of the abdominal muscles.

An important thing to remember while doing crunches is to keep your lower back pressed against the floor and to press your heels into the floor. This helps stabilize the lower body so you can concentrate on contracting only the abdominal muscles.

With your knees bent considerably to avoid strain on the lower back, slowly raise your head and shoulders off the floor and hold for a few seconds, then lower back down. Do not allow your chin to touch your chest because bending the head forward excessively in this position puts pressure on the neck and spinal cord. Instead, imagine that you are holding an apple under your chin as you rise up for every crunch.

If necessary, lightly place your hands on either side of your head for support on the way down. Never pull forward on your head as you crunch upward, however, since this puts unnecessary stress on the delicate tissues of the neck.

Try crossing your arms in front of your chest at first, and as you begin to fatigue, support your neck only if needed as you lower down. Since abdominal muscles (like calves) require high reps to see results, start out by doing as many crunches as you comfortably can. Ultimately, work your way up to sets of twenty-five or more, repeating until you have reached a goal of at least four sets.

To activate the oblique abdominal muscles, (especially the external oblique, which runs along the side and partly in the front of the torso), raise one shoulder to the opposite knee in a twisting motion while you are doing your crunches. You can perform your reps repeatedly doing one side at a time (for example, right elbow to left knee) or you can alternate sides (right elbow to left knee, return to starting position, then, left elbow to right knee).

How fast you will see results in your strength training program depends on many factors, including your genetic makeup, present physical condition, workout frequency, intensity, and consistency.

Allow time for your transformation to take place, and keep in mind that the changes occurring on the inside are just as important as the visible outward changes. You are embarking on an invigorating journey that will last the rest of your life. Take your time and savor every wonderful moment.

Dangerous Exercises

As a health care professional who has treated many patients with exercise induced symptoms throughout the years, I have found that performing certain popular, yet potentially dangerous, exercises and stretches is simply asking for trouble.

I have already warned you about some common weight training mistakes. Here are a few of the important floor exercises and stretches that you should avoid. I recommend that you never do deep knee bends where the thighs touch the lower legs. Not only can this exercise overstretch the ligaments of the knee, but it can irritate the delicate tissues that surround the knee joint. If you have ever had knee problems, you know how frustrating this can be, because pain and stiffness in your knees prevents you from doing practically everything you love to do.

Another no-no is the popular hurdler's stretch, in which you sit on the floor with one leg bent at an angle behind you and reach toward the other outstretched leg in the hurdler's position. Bending the knee at this angle puts a significant amount of abnormal stress on the knee joint. Cartilage and ligament damage are just a few of the possible soft tissue injuries associated with this stretch.

Instead, gently pull the leg in toward the groin area, not behind you at an angle. Stretch from this position, being careful not to overstretch or bounce. To extend the reach of your arms, you can wrap a towel around the foot of the outstretched leg, pulling gently, never to the point of pain.

I have often recommended yoga to my patients and friends over the years, for both the physical and mental benefits. Although most yoga postures are safe and effective, a popular yoga posture called the plough is potentially dangerous, especially for beginners. You may have seen this exercise on videos or in various exercise classes. The reason that I do not recommend this exercise is because of the stress that this position puts on the neck and the spinal tissues of the thoracic spine (or the area between your shoulder blades).

While performing the plough, the person doing this stretch lies flat on the floor, and then brings their legs all the way over their head and tries to touch the floor with their feet. Besides possibly overstretching ligaments, this position can adversely affect the spinal discs and nerves. No matter how flexible you may be, your neck and spinal column were not designed to withstand that particular kind of weight bearing pressure.

Also, if you have back problems, be particularly cautious of any exercise in which you lift both legs off the ground at the same time. Although some exercises involving this motion could possibly help strengthen the back, this exercise is potentially harmful if done improperly, or if you have a weak or damaged back.

I have already warned you not to do sit-ups or crunches pulling with your hands behind your neck, because of the strain it puts on the cervical vertebrae of the neck region. A better position is to cross your arms in front of your chest. Keeping your knees bent while doing crunches is imperative in order to avoid straining the back. When the legs are straight, there is tension on the hip flexing muscles, particularly the psoas major muscle, which attaches directly to the lumbar vertebrae of the lower back.

The same principle of keeping your knees bent during crunches holds true for standing straight leg toe touches. You probably remember this exercise from elementary school physical education classes. During this dangerous stretch, the exerciser stands up straight and then bends forward at the waist to see how far he can reach to the floor with his legs straight.

This is especially dangerous for people with lumbar (lower back) disc problems because it stresses the soft tissue of the lumbar region and can compress the sciatic nerve, which exits from the vertebrae in the lower back and runs down the back of the leg.

If you have ever experienced the excruciating pain of sciatica, you should remember not to do any kind of straight leg stretches. Ballet barre stretches are potentially dangerous for the same reason. Bouncing while in this position, trying to reach further, is asking for even more trouble. You should always keep your knees at least slightly bent while doing any type of stretches.

Similarly, when stretching the neck muscles, never use quick, jerky motions. Avoid extreme rotation, flexion, and extension of the head, which can damage the delicate cervical tissue, including nerves and discs.

Instead, slowly and gently stretch the neck side-to-side by bringing the ear toward the shoulder. This is much safer and more effective than the rapid rolling of the head in a circle. I literally cringe every time I see a boxer, football player, or other athlete quickly jerk their head from side to side or rapidly roll their head in a circle around their shoulders. Please refer to Chapter 36 for additional information about stretching the neck and upper back region.

The stretches and exercises listed above are simply a few of the ones that I personally find to be most disturbing. You will encounter many more along your

Pura Vida Path and hopefully be able to recognize them by using some of the anatomical and physiological information that you have accumulated on your own truth-seeking journey.

Perhaps the most important way to avoid physical injury and delays as you travel through life is to use the First Stepping Stone as a touchstone, listening to your body's built in warning signs and signals, and taking time to strengthen the connection between your physical body and your inner spirit.

As you have already found, taking time to slow down and quiet the extraneous stimuli surrounding you can help you make this connection and concentrate on your own personal goals. Whether those goals involve achieving optimal health or simply creating a more balanced, happier way of life, remember, you, and only you, have the power within you to make it happen. Dig deep!

On the Road

During certain phases of our lives when we were traveling frequently for business purposes, Len and I have spent more time flying, driving, or staying in hotels than in the comfortable sanctuary of our own home. Like most people, we sometimes find it very challenging to maintain consistent exercise and eating habits while traveling.

Fortunately, exercising regularly and eating well is fairly easy within the controlled environment of our peaceful home, yet there have been times when the momentum of our healthy routine was completely stalled by an unexpected business trip or extended vacation.

If your lifestyle involves frequent travel, you too, have likely found that being away from home presents its own unique set of challenges, in addition to exciting and interesting new experiences.

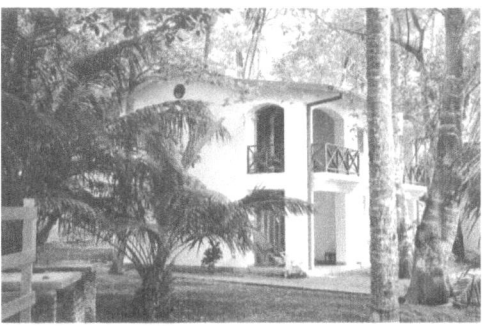

Like every other aspect of your personal Pura Vida journey, the secret to maintaining a healthy lifestyle while traveling away from home is simply a matter of proper balance. Although it is sometimes desirable to give yourself a little break from your normal routine, going to extremes by eating or doing anything you want can cause you to lose your healthy momentum, stumble off your path, and have difficulty finding your way again.

Since it is difficult to start rebuilding momentum from a dead stop, try not to let your Pure Energy Momentum in any aspect of your healthy lifestyle come to a screeching halt. It is much easier to reestablish your momentum by picking up from a pace that may be slower than normal, but is still moving on the right track.

One way to prevent temptation while traveling is to plan ahead. If we know that we are going to be staying at a hotel for more than a few days, we make a quick trip to the grocery or convenience store as soon as we get settled in. One of the first things that we usually purchase is a gallon or two of distilled water. Perhaps the most important item that you should have readily available while traveling is pure water.

On extended trips, we have learned to bring such survival basics as a few plastic bowls, cups, knives, forks, spoons, and of course, our trusty water bottles. It usually takes a few trips to establish your system, but you can do it with a little creative thinking.

If you are staying in a room without a small refrigerator or cooking burner, load up a small cooler with fresh fruits, lowfat breakfast and sports bars, and healthy dry goods. Traveling with these types of snacks allows you more control of what you eat, rather than forcing you to settle for what is available from restaurants, fast food stores, or even vending machines. Being prepared can also save you a considerable amount of money in the long run.

If you do have a small refrigerator, you can store healthy foods and drinks such as skim milk, juice, yogurt, and fruit. A healthy, whole-grain cereal can make a quick, nutritious breakfast or snack any time of the day. If your accommodations include a stovetop burner, oatmeal, soup, beans, and rice are just a few of your healthy eating options.

If you are staying at a hotel that has a gym, use it. Hotel gyms may not have all of your favorite equipment, but be creative and take advantage of whatever they do have to offer. No gym? Climb the stairs. If you climb stairs briskly for an extended period of time, you can efficiently work the large muscle groups of your buttocks and thighs.

To help counteract the hidden dietary fat that it is hard to avoid when traveling, and also to keep up your pure energy level, take a long walk or energizing run, or swim a few laps in the pool if one is available.

You may be surprised how much more enjoyable your trip is when you leave the comfort of your room and explore the area around you. Be adventurous and take advantage of any opportunity to spend time in the great outdoors, perhaps discovering a new energizing sport or activity that is entirely different than what you are accustomed to.

Back in your hotel room, try to keep up your energy level by doing some form of exercise regularly. Sit-ups, push-ups, calf raises, stretches, and lunges are a few of the exercises you can perform with only your bodyweight in the privacy of your home away from home. One of the awesome benefits of the Zoga stretching routine is that it was designed to be done anywhere and only takes ten to fifteen minutes, so if you do nothing else when traveling, take a few minutes to do your Zoga.

Remember the gallon of water you brought with you or purchased at the store? We have actually used ours as a weight for curls, triceps extensions, and other resistance exercises on occasion. It is not always easy, but if you really want to, you can find ways to maintain your high energy, healthy lifestyle under any conditions without losing your pure energy momentum.

Practical Advice

I have always believed that everything happens for a reason and that, in many cases, the reason is not immediately obvious. Sometimes it takes years for me to see why events transpired as they did at a particular time or stage in my own eventful journey through life. From the unique perspective of this point in my own Pura Vida Path, I can now see why my journey included many of the complicated twists and turns that were not part of my original plan, but instead part of a master plan that involved people from all over the world.

I truly feel that part of the reason that I became a chiropractor, treating and consulting thousands of patients and spending countless hours on my own truth seeking mission was so that I would obtain a sufficient level of experience and knowledge to help others on a broad scale through this book and related projects.

When I first began my formal education as an enthusiastic college student, fresh from my mountaintop home, my plan was much more naïve and simpler, in accordance with the world that I was living in at the time.

I had no idea that one day I would appear on international television or that hundreds of people from all over the world would ask me health related questions via electronic mail on a regular basis. Neither could I have predicted that I would sometimes struggle to make a conscious effort not to be constantly swept up in the somewhat frenetic pace of our modern world as it plunges into the unknown territory of the new millennium.

Some things never change, however. Throughout my own evolving Pura Vida Journey, I have found that what people do not know can truly hurt them and that most people benefit tremendously from everyday, practical advice and simple reminders.

The most common sense advice that has stood the test of time is usually the very information that helps us choose the next right step at precisely the right time. I sincerely hope that some of the following information and advice may help prevent you from suffering needlessly and perhaps even change your life.

If the subject in question form is not of particular interest to you at this point in your journey, please skim through it anyway and file it away for future reference, if needed. Here are the answers to some of the most practical questions that

I have been asked most frequently over the years. In addition, you will find additional current information and valuable advice by visiting www.pure-life.com at any time.

Q. *Why is sleeping on your stomach not good for your neck and back?*

A. There is no way to sleep on your stomach without putting some torque or twisting in your spine, especially in the neck region. This can be harmful to the spinal column because it puts pressure on the delicate spinal nerves over an extended period of time, and may result in stiffness, neck pain, and headaches.

The ideal position for sleeping is on your back, with a pillow under your neck to support the cervical curve. If you sleep on your side, try to switch sides frequently and position your pillow so that your head and neck are level with the bed and not tilted at an angle. Since there is less stress on the lower back when your legs are bent, try sleeping with a pillow under your knees if you are sleeping on your back, or between your knees if you sleep on your side.

The most important furniture investment you will ever make is buying a high quality mattress. Sleeping on a lumpy, saggy mattress for prolonged periods of time can cause serious musculoskeletal problems and result in a dramatic loss of energy.

Q. *What kind of pillow should I use?*

A. This is an important question since sleeping on a pillow that does not properly support your neck or causes it to tilt forward can gradually decrease the angle of the cervical curve and cause pain, stiffness and misalignment of the vertebrae over time.

There are three natural curves in the spine that naturally increase its strength and flexibility: the cervical curve in the neck, the thoracic curve in the mid back, and the lower back or lumbar curve. Just as the curve in a bridge or other structure increases its weight bearing capacity, so too, do the curves in your spine.

Loss of the cervical curve can be a result of overstretching of the ligaments, as is often seen after a serious car accident. This loss of curve can result in decreased weight bearing strength of the neck supporting the head and can cause pain and stiffness, possibly affecting vital nerve flow.

Sometimes it seems that I have been researching and searching for the perfect pillow for most of my adult life. There are a multitude of different types of cervical or neck pillows available on the market today. If you are like most people, you have tried at least a few different types, and hopefully found a pillow that you are comfortable with.

I personally have a stack of different pillows that I have given a chance and then thrown in the attic or given away. If you are still experimenting with different pillows, trying to find the perfect one, you may find the following information helpful.

As is often the case, the most expensive frequently advertised pillows aren't always the best ones. Some people swear by Tempurpedic or memory foam type pillows that are made of a foam type material that bounces back after applied pressure is removed. I know many people who are extremely particular about pillows who say that they can't sleep on anything but this type of pillow. A few people that I know prefer buckwheat filled pillows, but the noise they make as you are sleeping is annoying to some people.

Others prefer air or water filled pillows. The concept behind water based pillows is great, but many people find them to heavy or awkward to use. I'll probably always experiment with pillows searching for the ideal one. At present, my favorite pillow is one that wasn't even designed for sleeping, but rather for hugging or stress relief. Perhaps you have seen the lightweight, huggable, small roll shaped pillows covered in micro fiber type material and filled with tiny micro beads of polystyrene in drug stores or airport kiosks. I have several and prefer the more substantial higher quality versions. Since they are inexpensive, I simply buy a new one when the old one stretches out.

Also, feather pillows are ideal for providing support without being overly hard, and will conform to the contours of your neck more easily than a foam pillow. The problem with feather pillows, however, is that, often, they are simply too flat. If you are industrious, you can actually open up the seam and adjust the firmness by adding or removing more feathers until the pillow is more comfortable for you. You may even want to tie a ribbon around the middle to give it more of a butterfly shape. The procedure is a little messy, but many people have found it very effective.

The bottom line, in my opinion, is to use the first stepping stone once again and listen to the innate intelligence of your unique body rather than the marketing specialists on television.

Whenever possible, do not forget to take your most comfortable pillow with you when traveling, since hotel pillows are notoriously flat and hard, and often the cause of torticollis or stiffness in the neck region. I sometimes take a small pillow with me on extended airline flights along with a cozy scarf or wrap, since cold drafts (especially on planes and in hotel rooms) seem to frequently trigger stiff necks.

Q. *Why is prolonged sitting not good for your back?*

A. The human body was designed to walk or run for miles, not sit in chairs for prolonged periods of time. While sitting, there is more weight bearing pressure on the discs in your lower back than there is when standing or walking. When your body is in a reclining position, however, the weight bearing pressure is distributed more evenly throughout the spine.

Sitting is an inevitable part of today's lifestyle. There are some things you can do, however, to lessen the detrimental effects of prolonged sitting. While driving in a car or sitting for extended periods of time, be sure to maintain the lumbar curve of the spine by placing a pillow or lumbar support behind your back.

When driving, sit fairly close to the wheel with your knees bent. On long trips take some time to get out of the car and walk around, since it is much better to spend a few minutes stretching, than to spend weeks or months suffering with back pain or sciatica.

When sitting at a desk or at home, try to avoid slouching. Instead, sit straight and keep your feet flat on the floor whenever possible. Try to stand up and walk around as often as you can, even if it is only for a few minutes. The more you sit, the more you should walk to help counteract the negative effects of immobility and weight bearing pressure on your spinal column and lumbar discs.

Q. *What is the safest way to lift?*

A. Remember these three important words anytime you are lifting: Use Your Legs. Never bend straight forward from the waist without bending your knees, even if you are simply picking up a piece of paper. When your knees are bent, even slightly, it takes some of the strain off of your lower back.

Focus on keeping the object that you are lifting as close to your body as possible. Bend your knees and squat, keeping your back straight and your stomach muscles tight. Concentrate your energy on lifting with your strong thigh muscles, not your easily injured back muscles and surrounding delicate spinal tissues.

Move slowly and avoid sudden movements while lifting. Do not hold the load away from your body, and avoid twisting your torso while lifting at all costs. Instead, take small steps with your feet to position your body so that it is aligned with the object that you are lifting or setting down.

If you chose to wear a back support, please be aware that you may be tempted to lift more weight than usual while wearing one. Be cautious of becoming overly reliant on back supports and weight lifting belts. They may mask some of the muscular warning signs from your body and tempt you to push your back past its normal limits.

When carrying luggage or other bulky objects, always try to counterbalance the load by carrying something on each side. Do not throw everything over one shoulder and lean to the side. This can cause serious structural spinal problems over an extended period of time.

A backpack is ideal for balancing the load but can cause shoulder and nerve impingement problems if the weight is too heavy. Always use a trolley or wheeled luggage whenever possible, especially in airports and while walking for long distances in the city.

This is especially important to remember with schoolchildren who carry heavy books day after day, often altering the permanent structure of their delicate and growing spinal columns. There are several orthopedically designed backpacks that are helpful in properly distributing weight on children's shoulders. Some have adjustable air or thick cushioned padding in the straps or main body of the backpack.

Q. *My job involves standing on my feet all day. Is there anything I can do to make it easier on my lower back?*
A. If possible, stand with one foot up on a footrest and change positions frequently. Of course, wearing a comfortable shoe with good arch support makes a considerable difference.

Many people complain of back pain after shopping for hours in a mall or similar setting. Be aware that, unlike carpeted or wooden floors, concrete floors and cement sidewalks have absolutely no give.

The discs in your spine act as mini shock absorbers. Unfortunately, your vertebral discs and joints are compressed when you walk on hard surfaces or wear shoes with no cushion for extended periods of time.

No matter how much some women love the appearance of high-heeled shoes (myself included) they may find it necessary to limit the amount of time spent wearing them. The small joints, bones, and nerves of your feet can be damaged over time by being forced into an unnatural position, either by wearing a heel that is too high or by being squeezed into a shoe that is too pointy.

In addition, wearing high heels causes the pelvis to tilt at an unnatural angle, throwing off the foundation of the whole spine. If you must stand on your feet all day, follow the fourth stepping stone by respecting your body and taking care of your hard working feet.

Invest in a good pair of shoes or cushioned insoles and save the stylish, less comfortable and non-supportive shoes for short-term fun and special occasions. I have always had great luck with heavily cushioned, thick soled athletic shoes and frequently wear moccasin type shoes with contoured rubber insoles for absorbing shock when I know that I am going to be on my feet for extended periods.

The popular Croc clog type shoes that are sold widely are a comfortable shoe that doesn't stress the joints of the feet; however, the design can possibly create some instability of the knee joints when worn for long periods or worn while exercising.

Fortunately, even traditional men's dress shoes are being manufactured with more athletic heels and shock absorbing insoles, so shop around and keep trying until you find a shoe that is comfortable and offers extra support and cushioning.

Q. *My job involves sitting at a desk eight to ten hours a day. What can I do to make it more comfortable and safe?*

A. First of all, anyone who has to sit for such long periods should try to offset this inactivity with adequate amounts of exercise so that their body can function more efficiently.

Fortunately, there are a few things that you can do to take some of the risks out of an office job. Whenever possible, position yourself so that you are looking straight ahead and so your body is in a somewhat straight line with your work. Twisting just a few degrees may not seem harmful, but day after day, week after week, the negative effects can be cumulative and dramatic.

To reduce the risk of muscle strains, avoid leaning and reaching at extreme angles. Take time to organize your work area so that objects you use most are within easy reach. It is usually smarter to get up from your chair rather than reach across a long distance. Besides, it is much better for your back to get up and move around as often as possible.

When using a computer, always attempt to place the monitor directly in front of you. Your eyes should be level with the screen. Looking too far up or down for extended periods can cause problems ranging from muscular tension and spasm to headaches and neck and shoulder pain.

Invest in a good copyholder to avoid the neck strain caused by turning your head to one side. There are many options available, such as freestanding holders that clip to the monitor, and ones that tilt backward or swivel. Place the copyholder as close as possible to screen level.

Pay special attention to the lighting in the room. Eyestrain from even a small amount of glare can lead to headaches and neck and shoulder tension. Most computers have an anti-glare filter built in, but not all have anti radiation filters, which are a very good idea, especially if you spend a lot of time working on the computer.

It is essential that you have a good chair that supports your spine and allows proper blood and nerve flow to the lower extremities. An uncomfortable chair that does not fit your body properly can cause problems from the neck and arms all the way down to the lower back and legs.

Since we were all created with different shapes and sizes, it is necessary to try out many different chairs to find the one that is right for you. We recently spent close to an hour doing just that, playing musical chairs, much to the amusement of the store's salesperson.

Expensive, high back executive chairs are not ideal for doing deskwork for extended periods, although the neck support is helpful for leaning back on short breaks. As with everything else in an office setting, the more adjustable a chair is, the better chance you have of custom fitting it to your body.

Of course, proper posture is a necessity for anyone who sits for extended periods. Try to keep your feet flat on the floor and avoid slouching. Many chairs come with built in lumbar support, but frequently the added foam is still is not enough to fill in the space between your back and the chair.

An adjustable backrest can give your back even more support by placing the backrest exactly where you need it. You can also use lumbar pillows and cushions to support the lower back and make you more aware of your posture. You might want to experiment with different types of lumbar pillows or cushions, including the adjustable air or memory foam versions.

Look for a chair with a seat that supports approximately two-thirds of your thighs and slopes downward, allowing your hips to be higher than your knees. This position prevents the blood circulation from being cut off to your lower legs and feet. Make sure that the seat has adequate padding to help prevent loss of blood and nerve flow.

As I have often observed with my male patients, if a person walks or sits with a fat wallet in their back pocket, they can alter the foundation of their whole spine over time, resulting in significant lower back pain or discomfort. It is usually difficult for men to adjust to not carrying their wallet in their back pocket, but the ones that do almost always tell me what a difference it makes in their lower back pain.

One of the worst things that you can do to your neck is to hold the telephone on your upraised shoulder while you use the computer, type, or write. This repetitive type strain on the muscles and nerves of the cervical region can have serious consequences.

Phone accessories that raise the telephone to your ear help, but the muscles are still tensed and the neck is bent at an unnatural angle. Speakerphones are a much less dangerous option. Telephone headsets are ideal for someone who uses the phone regularly, and can literally save you a great deal of headache. The same holds true for mobile phones and blue tooth devices such as the Blackberry. If you frequently use a cell phone, a headset or speakerphone may reduce harmful radiation, as well.

Q. *Is there anything I can do to prevent the painful knots and spasms in my neck?*

A. There are a number of reasons why millions of people suffer from painful spasms and tension in the neck area. To find the cause of the problem, it is usually necessary to seek help from a qualified health care provider. Depending on the cause, there are a few things you can do at home to help relieve neck and shoulder pain or discomfort.

In the normal spine, there is a gentle C-shaped curve in the neck that allows you to look upward and that helps support the weight of the head. Often, this curve is flattened as a result of trauma, such as car accidents, during which the ligaments are overstretched or damaged. When this cervical curve is decreased or even reversed, it is much harder for the neck to hold up the heavy weight of the head. Also, the neck and shoulder muscles are placed under a great deal of stress, when there is a loss of the normal curve in the neck.

Continuous flexion of the neck (looking down) can also have a negative effect on the soft tissue and nerves of the neck and shoulder region. If your job involves constant flexion of the neck, it is imperative that you take frequent breaks to stretch your neck as often as possible. Without sufficient movement, over time, nerve supply flowing from the neck to the arms can be obstructed and lead to tingling or numbness in the arms and fingers and may eventually lead to headaches and other neurological symptoms.

Just as there is a continuous flow between the fluids on a cellular level, there is also a certain flow, similar to electricity, within the nervous system. Whenever there is an obstruction of the nerve flow, the part of the body that is supplied by that nerve does not function at its fullest potential.

One of the things that you can do to stimulate proper nerve flow is to obtain a sufficient amount of exercise. The lymphatic system and the digestive system function more efficiently with proper physical activity, and the nervous system is no exception.

Walking is a surprisingly good exercise for neck muscles, especially when you swing your arms. Swimming is wonderful because there is no weight bearing pressure on the joints and discs. Strengthening the muscles around the neck, including the traps and smaller spinal muscles also helps stabilize and support the neck and prevent pain and spasm.

As I stated earlier, you should never roll your head around quickly or jerk it from side to side. Avoid excessive rotation of the neck. It is better to laterally flex the neck by slowly, gently bringing the ear toward the shoulder and holding for a few seconds. You can also help strengthen the muscles by applying gentle resistance against a towel stretched across the forehead, back and sides of the head. Never strain or take a stretch to a point where there is discomfort.

You can stretch the trapezius muscles (traps) by simply dropping your arms to your sides and slowly rolling your shoulders in a circular motion. By gradually adding light hand weights, the muscles become stronger. Strong muscles reinforce the joints, and the neck consists of many joints between the individual vertebrae. Trap shrugs involve the motion of simply shrugging, or bringing both shoulders toward the ears. This exercise can be done with or without dumbbells. Trap shrugs are particularly good for strengthening the upper trapezius muscle, which runs between the neck and the shoulders.

A good way to break up the spasm cycle often related to stress and tension is to take a few moments to relieve the neck and the rest of the spine of its constant weight bearing responsibility by simply lying down.

When you are in a reclining position, the weight bearing pressure is distributed more evenly throughout your body and there is less direct pressure on specific vertebrae and discs. By placing a cervical roll or medium sized, rolled up towel under your neck, you help to relax the neck and shoulder muscles.

Taking just a few minutes from your day to rest in this position will also support the cervical curve, and increase nerve supply and blood flow. Not only will you be breaking up the cycle of spasm by not allowing the tension to build, but you will often have the added benefits of more energy and better powers of concentration.

Q. *Are there any safe and effective self care products that you can recommend for neck and back pain?*

A. Many years ago, one of my patients asked me an interesting question. They said, "Out of all of the products that you have recommended over the years for neck and back pain, if you had to pick just one, what would it be?" Without hesitation, my answer was "The Backnobber."

The official name for this durable, S shaped, self care massage tool with small knobs on either end is the Original Backnobber 2 and it is manufactured by a sincere company called the Pressure Positive Company. It is engineered to be a comfortable extension of your own hands, allowing you to apply direct, localized pressure on painful, tight, knots and spasms in your muscles in those hard to get areas that you simply can't reach on your own.

To find out more, visit the manufacturer's comprehensive, information based website: www.pressurepositive.com. Here, you can preview parts of the thirty-five page, fully illustrated backnobber user guide that comes with each backnobber. You can also learn about trigger point therapy and find out exactly how to use this awesome tool to alleviate muscle pain due to causes such as injuries, stress, bad postural habits and overuse.

This ergonomically designed deep muscle massage tool uses leverage so you don't need strength or stamina to press deeply into your muscles to manage trigger point flare-ups. This direct pressure on specific points in muscles of the neck, shoulder blades, and lower back relaxes the muscles and brings blood flow and oxygen to the affected area, breaking the cycle of spasm.

Using both hands, simply put a knob on the painful spot and push out on the end facing your front to apply as much pressure as you need to relax the tense, knotted muscle. One of the things that I particularly like about the backnobber is that you can use your backnobber anywhere, anytime, without having to wait for an appointment.

In addition to the Backnobber, another of my all time favorite products for relieving minor muscular aches and pains is a high quality digital moist heating pad that can be purchased at most medical supply stores or online. I like the brands that cost a little more and have covers that attract moisture as opposed to the less expensive, drug store brands that utilize a piece of foam type fabric that must be moistened before using.

The higher quality moist heating pads are also more flexible and conform to the joints and curves of the body. If you have any doubt whether you should be using heat or ice for a specific condition, please ask your physician or primary health care provider.

Q. *I really want to quit smoking and cut back on drinking. Any advice?*
A. One of the best ways to eliminate negative addictions, such as cigarette smoking or alcohol abuse, is to replace them with positive habits such as exercise, meditation, or outdoor activities that you truly enjoy. Remember, positive change in one area can have a domino effect on all other parts of your life.

Knowing the facts sometimes makes it easier to choose the direction in which you want your life to continue. For example, if you are a heavy drinker, it may help motivate you to cut back or quit by realizing that you are increasing your risk not only of liver cirrhosis, but also of cancer of the oral cavity, larynx, and esophagus. Some evidence also suggests that regular alcohol consumption increases breast cancer risk in women.

Also, simply knowing that nine out of ten men who die from lung cancer smoke cigarettes should be reason enough for anyone who smokes to stop now. Not smoking helps prevent many diseases, not only lung cancer. According to the American Cancer Society, three out of four men who get any kind of cancer smoke cigarettes.

In order to turn negative habits into positive ones, try to surround yourself with healthy people and do not be afraid of being a little different from the norm. It may take some time for people to adjust to the changes you have made, but ultimately they will respect you even more for it and someday, they may even ask your advice on making healthy lifestyle changes.

Creating Health

As you have probably noticed, one of the key words throughout this book is prevention. The old Ounce of Prevention principle applies not only in everyday situations such as working, lifting, and exercise, but also in less obvious areas such as stress reduction, posture, and breathing.

You now have the powerful, life changing information that you need to help prevent cancer, cardiovascular conditions, and a long list of diseases. You also possess knowledge that can help you create a healthier lifestyle and increase your pure energy level. Only you can transform that information and knowledge into dynamic actions in your daily lifestyle that will significantly improve the quality of your health and, in turn, each and every day of the rest of your life.

And finally, remember, nothing has more power over your body than your mind. Recent research verifies something that most of us have always believed. Positive thinking, faith, and prayer can improve the quality of your health and speed up recovery time, in addition to many other life changing effects.

Personally, I try to make it a point to start every day with quiet time for meditation and prayer, concentrating on everything that I have to be grateful for and asking God for guidance. I have found that when I take this time out, my days are much more productive and creative and my goals and intentions are much clearer.

As you are creating a healthier lifestyle by incorporating meditation and quiet time for reflection into your daily lifestyle, you may find that it is easier to tap into your artistic or creative energy. This exciting, stimulating force often lies dormant during times of stress.

By taking a little time to experiment with your own unique form of creative expression, you can actually decrease the stress and tension in your life. You can also activate phenomenal new, untapped energy that will help you get through the day and increase your productivity in other areas, such as work and relationships.

Since I was a child, I have always loved making things with my hands, and have experimented with practically every artistic medium available. I have found that my Pura Vida Journey involves a great deal of creative expression and that my life is much fuller when I am actively involved in some artistic endeavor.

I also believe that everyone has some creative talent and that expressing that inner creativity enhances the state of one's health and well-being. Do not block your pure energy by being afraid to march to the beat of a different drummer. Be bold. Color outside the lines and remember, when you are allowing your creative energy to flow, there are no rules!

It appears that I am not alone in my love of art and creative expression, since the Pura Vida Trailblazers and other wise souls have been making the world a more beautiful place for thousands of years. Keep the images of creativity that appeal most to you in mind as you uncover and utilize the sixteenth stepping stone (the last but certainly not the least along your pathway).

Stepping Stone # 16: *Explore your creative potential and boldly express your artistic energy in a way that is uniquely right for you.*

As you have already experienced from utilizing Stepping Stone #10, another spoke in the wheel of optimal health is spending quality time in nature. Taking time out of your busy day to connect with the earth increases your positive energy level and helps you to become a healthier, more joyful person.

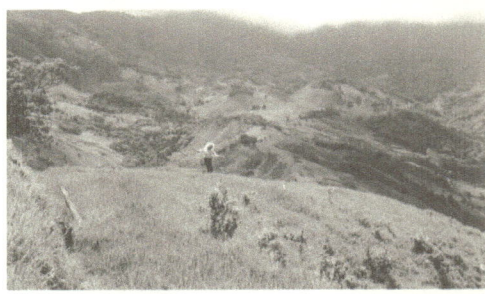

If you have felt a deep longing in your soul for something more meaningful, take some time and get out where you can put your worries on the back burner, stretch your legs, and breathe fresh air. Feel the wind in your face, the sand between your toes and the sun caressing your shoulders as you mountain bike, run on the beach, or take a brisk walk around your neighborhood. Lie in the snow and gaze at the clouds.

Get outside and allow yourself to experience a meaningful, deep connection with the earth, even if it means taking off your shoes and walking in the grass on your lunch break. Take just a moment to truly live in the moment.

Now that you are nearing the end of this stage of your personal, allegorical Pura Vida journey, let's take a few minutes to contemplate just how far you have come since you took those first few steps in the right direction toward creating optimal health and changing your life for the better.

Perhaps the most important step you took was the first one, which became your touchstone and the foundation on which you built your permanently healthier lifestyle. By using Stepping Stone # 1 and listening closely to the innate intelligence of your body while letting your soul be your guide, you connected with your inner energy and gained a sturdy, reliable anchor in rough weather and unknown waters.

As a result of connecting with your innate intelligence, you were able to fully utilize the power of the second crucial stepping stone along your Pure Life path by making a conscious effort to prevent and reduce the negative effects of stress in your daily life.

As you confidently continued along your unique path, you discovered that the third helpful stepping stone along your own unique path, consistent deep diaphragmatic breathing, is a vital component of your energizing Pura Vida Lifestyle.

At this point in your journey, you began to see that all of the Stepping Stones are interrelated and you began to feel the cumulative power of each step as you continued in the direction that you were meant to move in. You also recognized that there is a powerful force in the world much bigger than yourself, which connects us all to each other and to our fragile environment.

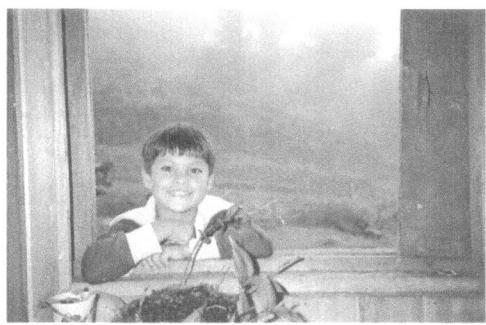

As your mental and physical muscles grew stronger and your senses became more acute, you also grew in awareness by using the fourth stepping stone, fully respecting and loving your body exactly as it is in each and every moment of your life. You realized that in every precious moment, you live and move in the presence of a higher power that gives you strength and energy when you are open to the life-affirming, spiritual energy of the universe.

In utilizing Stepping Stone #5, you began to integrate the Pure Energy Balance Principle into your daily lifestyle, balancing your Energy Input from high quality sources with your Energy Output, resulting in a stronger, healthier body, mind and spirit.

As a natural consequence of the building positive momentum of the previous five stepping stones, you easily found the sixth helpful stepping stone in achieving the healthy lifestyle you deserve by hydrating and nourishing your body with plenty of pure, fresh water throughout your Pura Vida journey.

As you rapidly grew in knowledge and awareness, Stepping stone # 7 (eating for the nutritional value of your food and not simply for instant gratification) became a natural, instinctive part of your daily lifestyle and nutritional choices.

Stepping Stone # 8, maintaining a strong, steady, pure momentum, came to you easily as you continued to grow in understanding and applied what you learned one step at a time, one day at a time. In providing fuel for your voyage, you discovered the intrinsic value of the ninth stepping stone, and found that the source and quality of your nutrients is equally as important as the amounts.

Not only did you increase the level of your energy by improving the quality of your physical fuel, but you also created a higher state of spiritual and emotional health, by using the tenth stepping stone, spending as much quality time in Nature as possible, connecting with your life force and breathing deeply.

As your journey progressed, you also focused your awareness and your mental energy on learning more about supplementation and utilizing Stepping Stone #11, supplementing your healthy diet with high quality vitamins and minerals when necessary.

Due partially to the added energy boost from more nutritious fuel sources gained as a result of applying the knowledge gained from the previous stepping stones, Stepping Stone # 12 brought an unprecedented level of strength, both inner and physical. Taking time to make exercise and physical activity a consistent, integral part of your high-energy lifestyle by using this twelfth helpful tool was even more rewarding and satisfying than you anticipated.

You discovered the valuable, life changing lesson of Flexible Strength while standing confidently on Stepping Stone # 13, including a regular program of stretching into your daily lifestyle. The simple stretching exercises that you learned helped you uncover hidden strengths and preventative health benefits that were surprisingly profound and significant.

You were finally able to unleash your full potential by consistently using the next two stepping stones; Stepping Stone #14, (including consistent aerobic exercise in your everyday Pura Vida Lifestyle) and Stepping stone # 15, (strengthening the muscles and bones of your body with the use of resistance or weights on a regular basis).

As you approached your intended destination in your newly strengthened body, more aware and informed than at any other time in your life, you uncovered and took advantage of the sixteenth stepping stone, along your pathway, exploring your creative potential and fully expressing your artistic energy.

As a result of your ongoing, ever changing Pura Vida journey, you have become like the exotic wild bird that Abeulo breathed Pure Life into. You have risen above the entanglements and complications of everyday life and found within yourself a limitless source of potential energy and strength.

Regardless of the everyday challenges facing you in your life, you know that you always have the power to change it for the better, simply by taking the next right step. Congratulations! You truly have created a healthier, more energetic lifestyle and improved the quality of your life and of your future. You are the master of your own destiny.

> *Live with intention. Walk to the edge. Listen hard.*
> *Practice wellness. Play with abandon. Laugh.*
> *Choose with no regret. Continue to learn.*
> *Appreciate your friends. Do what you love.*
> *Live as if this is all there is.*
>
> *Maryanne Rodmaches-Hershery*

Pura Vida!

Collectively, across the planet, we are all only just beginning to understand how intertwined our physical, mental, and spiritual aspects are. These boundaries are not as distinct as was once believed. As I wrote earlier, "Health is an optimum state of physical, mental, spiritual, and social well being."

In documenting my own version of the truth about optimal health while writing this book, I hope that I have provided you with some reassurance that you are not alone in your journey through life. I also hope that my research and words have provided you with some knowledge that will help you gain the confidence to make the right decisions in your daily life, and motivate you to keep moving consistently in the right direction.

No matter how slow your progress may seem at times, do not lose sight of your well-thought-out goals and highest intentions. As you travel along your unique path, take time to appreciate and enjoy the panoramic view along the way. Slow down and savor the feeling of become stronger, healthier, and more alive.

When your intentions are clear and focused, and you trust the intuitive part of your nature, making daily decisions and choices comes much easier. Your newly transformed lifestyle leads to a release of new energy, a joyous new life.

I have found that my life seems to flow most smoothly when I am open to new ideas and change. Achieving and maintaining good health does require discipline and focus, but it does not have to be boring. It can and should be an energizing and revitalizing adventure, to be enjoyed and savored every step of the way.

We have all experienced times in our lives when everything seems to come together—moments of clarity when everything clicks and you feel as if you are flowing with the natural course of events, doing exactly what you are meant to be doing at that particular point in time. Short lived as these moments may be, they are important because they give us hope and faith that there is a light at the end of the tunnel, that there is more to life than simply surviving or just getting by.

When you stop and take time to count your blessings, you realize that your health is the most precious gift of all. Without your health, it is difficult to fully enjoy success, accomplishments, and all of the wonderful kinds of love that the world has to offer.

When you focus on improving the quality of your health, you will find that those Pura Vida moments where everything seems crystal clear are a more frequent part of your life. When something makes sense to you and you truly believe it, keep applying it in your daily life, until it becomes a part of your overall lifestyle.

By making the right decisions and maintaining a healthy balance between your mind, body, and soul, you can create an inner reservoir of strength and peace that you can always return to and draw from in times of need.

And finally, remember, even when your life is at its most challenging, there is an incredible energy within you, keeping you alive. It is the same life force that, in the past, has energized, inspired, and uplifted you. That awesome force is always there—pure energy, pure life, Pura Vida!

The End

The Pure Life Stepping Stones

Stepping Stone #1: Listen closely to the innate intelligence of your body and let your soul be your guide.

Stepping Stone #2: The second crucial stepping stone along your Pure Life path is to make a conscious effort to prevent and reduce the negative effects of stress in your daily life.

Stepping Stone #3: Consistent deep diaphragmatic breathing is a vital component of the Pura Vida lifestyle, and is the third helpful stepping stone along your own unique path.

Stepping Stone #4: Respecting and loving your body exactly as it is at this moment is the fourth stepping stone on your Pura Vida journey.

Stepping Stone #5: Integrate the Pure Energy Balance Principle into your daily lifestyle.

Stepping Stone #6: Drinking plenty of pure water is the sixth helpful stepping stone in achieving the healthy lifestyle you deserve.

Stepping Stone #7: Eat for the nutritional value of your food, not simply for instant gratification.

Stepping Stone #8: Maintaining a strong, steady, pure momentum is the eighth stepping stone along your personal path.

Stepping Stone #9: Keep in mind that the source and quality of your nutrients is equally as important as the amounts.

Stepping Stone #10: Spend as much quality time in Nature as possible, connecting with your life force and breathing deeply.

Stepping Stone #11: Supplement your healthy diet with high quality vitamins and minerals.

Stepping Stone #12: Taking time to make exercise and physical activity a consistent, integral part of your high energy lifestyle is the twelfth Stepping stone along your path.

Stepping Stone #13: Including a regular program of stretching into your daily lifestyle is the powerful yet simple thirteenth stepping stone.

Stepping Stone #14: Include consistent aerobic exercise in your everyday Pura Vida Lifestyle.

Stepping Stone #15: Strengthen the muscles and bones of your body with the use of resistance or weights on a regular basis.

Stepping Stone #16: Explore your creative potential and boldly express your artistic energy.

978-0-595-45484-6
0-595-45484-4